MISSIONARY FITNESS

PREPARE YOUR
BODY & SPIRIT
FOR SERVICE

CALVIN BUHLER

Visit us at www.missionaryfitness.com

ISBN: 978-0-615-40021-1

Missionary Fitness is intended for healthy adults, age 18 and over. The advice and recommendations presented in this book are intended as informational and educational resources only. This book is not intended to replace the advice of a mission president, priesthood leader, medical or healthcare professional. Please consult a medical or healthcare professional before you begin any new exercise, nutrition, or supplementation program. The author and publisher disclaim any liability arising from directly or indirectly using this book and the information it contains.

PRAISE FOR MISSIONARY FITNESS

"I wish I had *Missionary Fitness* when I served my mission!"
-Robert G. Allen | Best-Selling Author

"The principles taught in *Missionary Fitness* helped me to lose 60 pounds in 6 months. I look great, but more importantly I feel great. This information changed my mission and literally saved my life."
-Elder Ryan Braschko | UT-SLC Mission

"*Missionary Fitness* is a break-through book unlike any other and will prove to be an effective and popular complement to every missionary's library. It's the only comprehensive resource to address the spiritual and physical needs of full-time missionaries. It's a must-read for all missionaries who want to prepare their body and spirit for service."
-Gregory Buhler, D.O. | Family Practice Doctor

"*Missionary Fitness* clearly illustrates the importance of physical health for missionaries and how it integrates with the spiritual dimension as well. After reading *Missionary Fitness* I wished this book had been available when I served my mission. My missionary experience and life since would have been healthier and happier."
-Elder Don Ziegler | LDS Church Employee
Wellness Coordinator

"To call this book refreshing, different, and better is an understatement that shows my weakness for language. I believe that any person who prayerfully studies and uses the principles taught in this book will transform their life both physically and spiritually. They will embody the physical representation of our spiritual potential and be a beacon of our Heavenly Fathers' love to the world."

-Neil Anderson | Radio Talk Show Host

"*Missionary Fitness* will radically transform your missionary experience. Based on eternal principles, it will guide you in unleashing your brilliance as a full-time missionary by aligning your body, mind, and spirit. In my experience it will prepare you for service better than any other book – outside of the scriptures."

-Garrett J. White | Author and Speaker

ACKNOWLEDGMENTS

Everyone, I believe, has a profound book idea hidden deep within the consciousness of their mind. The idea for such a book is based on some morsel of information unique to their own knowledge and experience. For unto whom much is given, much is required (see Luke 12:48). With such knowledge and experience comes great responsibility, even a divine stewardship to share with others so they may be lifted up and inspired to be more, do more, and ultimately have more. If this knowledge and experience touches at least one soul, how great shall be the joy of the one sharing the message.

I wouldn't have been able to share my message without the help and support of many people. I would first like to express my deepest gratitude and sincere appreciation to my Father in Heaven who is the source of all information and who has allowed me the privilege to be the vessel in delivering the information contained in this book. I would also like to thank my beautiful wife, Katie and my precious children, who sacrificed many things and selflessly endured the process of creating a book so I may get this message out.

Gratitude and appreciation also goes to: My mom, Debbie, for faithfully raising a "Stripling Warrior," for teaching me how to serve others and also for editing early copies of this manuscript. My dad, Greg, for supporting me on my mission and for showing me that nothing can stand in the way of achieving your dreams. My brother, David, for being a remarkable example to me in serving the Lord, which gave me the strength and courage to go on my mission, also for providing me with powerful insights and critical feedback on the information in this book.

My two mission presidents and their wives; President Richard G. Hinckley and Sister Jane Hinckley and President J. Richard Thorderson and Sister Thorderson. President Hinckley, thank you for believing in me enough to give me the opportunity to serve in the capacities I did and for having love and mercy on me despite my weaknesses. To all of my missionary companions and my missionary brothers (you know who you are), thanks for providing inspiration and support to me as we served together.

A big thanks to Heather Sachs for the front cover design and the interior layout, to Matt Stone for all the great photographs in this book and on the cover, and to Sam Allen who was the model for all the exercise photos.

Although I have only acknowledged a few names, many more individuals have had a hand in the creation of this book as they have helped me become the person I am today. Each one of you has left a positive mark on my life forever. For that I am eternally grateful and indebted. May I be blessed with the privilege of serving all of you the rest of my days.

Dedicated to my wife Katie,
whose missionary spirit brought us together!

TABLE OF CONTENTS

PREFACE

The idea for this book goes back several years to the time I was preparing for my mission. I had just finished a very successful collegiate athletic career and was in the best shape of my life. As an athlete I was naturally concerned with my level of health and fitness. In fact, from the time I was a young child, when I first began participating in sports, exercise and nutrition had become a way of life.

As the time approached to send in the application to go on my mission, my priorities began shifting. The focus of my life had changed from strengthening my physical body to strengthening my spirit. Of course, all my life I had been indirectly preparing for my mission by doing all the necessary things young men are instructed to do to prepare for a mission. I attended seminary and institute, church meetings and firesides, and studied the scriptures and prayed. But the time had come to be more focused and committed to directly preparing for my mission.

I was fortunate because my brother had just come home from his mission and we had an agreement - he would help me prepare for my mission and I would help him readjust to regular life. We did our best to live the missionary lifestyle while not actually being on a mission. We would get up early and go to bed early, we prayed and studied together, we read from the Missionary Guide, studied the discussions, and yes, we even role-played common missionary scenarios.

All of this preparation proved to be beneficial, but as I studied and prepared spiritually, I still felt like something was missing from the missionary lifestyle. I quickly realized the physical preparation of a missionary was just as important as the spiritual preparation. Missionaries are instruments in God's hands, but are limited by physical bodies. The spirit of a missionary may be willing but if the flesh is weak, a missionary may not reach his full potential.

As an athlete and having had extensive education in health, nutrition, and human performance, I was naturally concerned about the lack of exercise and quality of nutrition a typical missionary experiences prior to and during a mission. The Missionary "White" Handbook at the time instructed missionaries to "...schedule time to exercise regularly" (*Missionary Handbook*, 17). However, on the previous page, the recommended daily schedule outlines what a missionary should be doing every hour and half hour of the day with no mention of exercise. How was a missionary expected to "schedule time to exercise regularly" when there was no time allotted for it? Fortunately, the recommended daily schedule for missionaries has changed and now allocates 30 minutes each morning (except Sunday, of course) to exercise.

Health and fitness had become a way of life for me and I was willing to sacrifice it if necessary, to serve the Lord. However, I knew there had to be a way to incorporate health and fitness into the missionary lifestyle because a healthy missionary is a better instrument in the Lord's hands. This would require a regular exercise program and a good nutritional plan. So my search began for an exercise and nutrition program designed specifically for missionaries and their unique circumstances. I read every missionary preparation book, every talk by former and current prophets and General Authorities, every church manual, book, or other related resource I could find on missionary preparation and missionary service. When my exhaustive research was complete, I was disappointed. I found nothing with any real substance relating to the physical aspects involved with preparing for and serving a mission. Sure, the subject of physical fitness, health, and nutrition for missionaries was addressed but only to a small degree. The limited amount of information that did exist merely mentioned the importance of exercise and nutrition, but failed to explain how to prepare in this manner and then how to integrate it into the missionary lifestyle.

Unfortunately, no single resource with this important information existed for missionaries when preparing for and serving a mission. I sensed a real need for such a resource. At that moment, I made the decision to write a book explaining, in detail, how a missionary could incorporate health, fitness, and nutrition into their daily schedule so they could prepare for and serve to their full potential.

The inspiration for such a resource was reinforced many times while on my mission and over the years since returning home. I saw firsthand how small lifestyle changes prior to leaving on a mission and while serving could dramatically improve a missionary's ability to serve. After implementing the strategies and principles contained in this book prospective and full-time missionaries everywhere have radically changed their missions and their lives.

As a result, I have created a unique and powerful resource for current and future missionaries, which they can use to prepare their bodies and spirits for serving the Lord. My prayer for everyone who reads this book is that they may feel better, look better, have more confidence, and ultimately, be a better instrument in the Lord's hands.

– Calvin Buhler

SECTION I:

PREPARING FOR
MISSIONARY
FITNESS

INTRODUCTION:
"The Greatest Work in All the World"

Before his ascension into heaven for the last time, at the conclusion of his mortal ministry in Jerusalem, Jesus Christ appeared to his apostles with one final word of instruction. He said, "Go ye into all the world, and preach the gospel to every creature" (Mark 16:15). Surely, this was an extremely important message since it was the last one Jesus left with His most faithful followers. The importance of this message has continued in modern times as well (see D&C 68:8). Many prophets, ancient and modern, have emphasized the importance of missionary work. President Ezra Taft Benson said, "To faithful missionaries everywhere...go forward with faith and courage. You are engaged in the greatest work in all the world—the saving of the souls of the children of men. In this great work we cannot fail" (Benson, Conference Report, 129; emphasis added).

More recently, President Gordon B. Hinckley addressed a congregation at the homecoming of a recently returned mission president. He said, "Missionary work is the single most important work we can do in the Church"

(Hinckley, July 2004). The peaceful message of the gospel is needed in this world more than ever before, and God's kingdom on earth will continue to grow as a result of the nearly 60,000 faithful missionaries responding to the same instruction the Lord gave His apostles in Jerusalem.

It is an exciting time to be a missionary and to be involved with missionary work! Missionary work is constantly growing and evolving as the Church continues to mature as a worldwide organization with a vast international presence. Teaching and training methods are improving, daily schedules are adjusting, and study routines are being refined, all in an effort to better communicate the message of the gospel while more fully utilizing the Spirit.

There is something special that comes from sharing the Gospel of Jesus Christ with others. You will have the opportunity to participate with God in fulfilling His work and His glory, which is "to bring to pass the immortality and eternal life of man" (Moses 1:39). You are engaged in the Lord's work. You are on His errand and you are an instrument in His hands teaching His gospel to all who will listen.

The gospel message has a powerful impact on those who receive it as well as those who share it. Imagine how precious everyone with whom you share it is to Heavenly Father (see D&C 18:10). In exchange for your diligent service, you will be rewarded and richly blessed. Jesus said, "and if it so be that you should labor all your days in crying repentance unto this people, and bring, save it be one soul unto me, how great shall be your joy with him in the kingdom of my Father" (D&C 18:15).

Serving a mission will be rewarding but also challenging. You will be stretched physically, mentally, spiritually, and emotionally. You will grow and mature. You will learn the importance of the gospel in your life as well as in the lives of others. You will be involved with something bigger than yourself. You will learn to focus more on the things that really matter in life. You will have the opportunity to serve others, which is one of the greatest privileges our Father in Heaven can trust us with.

Missionary work is just that – a privilege. President Kimball said, "It is a great privilege to go on a mission... [you] must be physically well [and] spiritually well... I am asking for missionaries who have been carefully indoctrinated and trained through the family and organizations of the Church and who come to the mission with a great desire. I am asking...that we train prospective missionaries much better, much earlier, much longer, so that each anticipates his [or her] mission with great joy" (Kimball, 7-8).

Church leaders are re-emphasizing the fact that a mission is a privilege and you must be qualified to serve the Lord. Elder M. Russell Ballard said, "What we need now is the greatest generation of missionaries in the history of the Church. We need worthy, qualified, spiritually [and physically] energized missionaries...We don't need spiritually weak and semi-committed young men. We don't need you to just fill a position; we need your whole heart and soul. We need vibrant, thinking, passionate missionaries who know how to listen to and respond to the whisperings of the Holy Spirit. This isn't a time for spiritual weaklings" (*Ensign*, Nov. 2002: 47).

Due to the challenging nature of a mission, bishops and stake presidents are instructed to only recommend "those young men and women whom [they] judge to be spiritually, physically, mentally, and emotionally prepared to face today's realities of missionary work" (*Ensign*, Nov. 2002: 48). Aspiring young missionaries are taught and prepared spiritually, mentally, and socially from an early age. They are instructed and encouraged to read scriptures, pray, attend church meetings, go to seminary and institute, and participate in youth and other social activities. Despite this thorough preparation and training, most missionaries are still not progressing as much as they possibly can because one essential element is often neglected. The physical element is a crucial, but unfortunately, overlooked factor in preparing for and serving a mission.

Physical preparation is vitally important because missionary work is very demanding. It presents many unique challenges and experiences that are new and even foreign to most. It will test you in all areas of your life, especially physically. Missionaries are constantly on the go all day, everyday without much rest. The daily schedule is very intense, even for the most physically prepared. Missionaries are required to get up early and go without rest until late at night. It is difficult to eat a healthy diet because the busy schedule does not always permit the time to prepare nutritious meals and snacks.

The very nature of missionary work, although fun and exciting, is extremely stressful on the physical body. The stress weakens the immune system and tests the body's adaptive mechanisms leaving it vulnerable to fatigue, illness, and injury. A tired, sick, or injured missionary is not as effective at spreading the gospel as a healthy one. Living a healthy, active lifestyle enables the body to effectively handle stress, thus reducing the chance of illness and injury. Your level of health and fitness prior to and while serving a mission may propel you to success or stop you in your tracks!

Unlike other areas of missionary preparation, there are virtually no resources available to help missionaries prepare physically for their mission and maintain it throughout their service. This book has been written to provide that necessary resource. All the information you need is here – the expert advice, the practical wisdom, and the scientifically proven strategies.

This book will challenge, encourage, and teach you many things. You will be challenged to consider God's words in scriptures and through His prophets, regarding your health and fitness. You will be encouraged by the discovery of simple, yet practical strategies to maximize your physical and spiritual health while preparing for and serving your mission. You will learn why Jesus is the perfect example for both spiritual and physical health. You will learn what to pack for your mission in order to meet your health needs and fitness goals. You will learn nutritional strategies that will assist you in following a healthy eating plan. You will learn that fasting is as much a physical law as it is a spiritual law. You will learn important strategies to integrate proper exercise into your daily schedule. You will be given a complete exercise program tailored to the unique missionary lifestyle. You will learn the importance of proper rest and relaxation. You will learn how to recognize and avoid the common obstacles and pitfalls to Missionary Fitness success. You will learn all of this and much, much more.

Once you turn the page and begin reading the first chapter, your journey of physical and spiritual transformation will begin, and you will be on your way to physically qualifying for the privilege of participating in "the greatest work in all the world."

JESUS,
THE PERFECT EXAMPLE

The basic philosophy of a missionary is to serve God "with all your heart, might, mind, and strength" (see D&C 4:2). The packet you received announcing your mission call included a letter that states, "You have been recommended as one worthy to represent the Lord as a minister of the restored gospel...As such, you will be expected to maintain the highest standards of conduct and appearance."

As a missionary, you are a literal representative of the Lord and Savior, Jesus Christ. You are His personal messenger, delivering His message to those prepared to hear and receive it. To bear the responsibility of such a message, you must be prepared just as Jesus was when He first delivered the gospel message over two-thousand years ago. You should strive to pattern your life after the manner of Jesus, just as He commanded us to do when He said, "What manner of men [and women] ought ye to be? Verily I say unto you, even as I am" (3 Nephi 27:27).

Most missionaries have a strong desire to be like Jesus in every way and to live a life that exemplifies His life and teachings. They want to live as He lived, teach as He taught, preach as He preached, pray as He prayed, love as He loved, and obey as He obeyed. They want to follow in His every footstep. To fully be like Jesus means embracing how He lived. In order to emulate His life, you must first learn and understand how He lived and prepared for His mortal ministry.

Over two-thousand years have passed since Jesus walked the earth as a mortal man and we have primarily been taught to think of Him in a spiritual way. Many things have been written in the scriptures and in history books about Him as our spiritual leader, the Son of God, and the Savior of the world, but what about the other areas of His life? How was He prepared mentally, physically, spiritually, and socially for the ultimate ministry which ended in His crucifixion and reawakened with His resurrection?

Very little evidence of Jesus' early years and how He prepared for His ministry seem to exist. Observations from initial reading of the scriptures do not seem to share insights on this part of His life. However, we learn from a single verse of scripture in the Gospel of Luke the formula of how Jesus lived and prepared for His divine calling: "And Jesus increased in wisdom [mentally] and stature [physically], and in favour with God [spiritually] and man [socially]" (Luke 2:52). This simple verse tells us that, from an early age, Jesus grew and developed mentally, physically, spiritually, and socially.

Although the scriptures do not come right out and tell us the details of what Jesus did to grow and develop, we can come to a very accurate conclusion about the life of Jewish people and Jesus during that era by applying the written word of ancient and modern prophets, examining what Jesus taught through word and deed, and studying the anthropological and cultural information available.

Just as Jesus' preparation began long before the start of His mortal ministry, your preparation should begin before you receive your mission call. Elder David A. Bednar of the Quorum of the Twelve Apostles said, "The single most important thing you can do to prepare for a call to serve is to become a missionary long before you go on a mission" (*Ensign*, Nov. 2005: 45). To be completely ready for service, consider how you can prepare in the same manner as Jesus, so you can be a worthy representative of Him.

MENTAL PREPARATION

Jesus attended school at the local synagogue where He was mentored by a schoolmaster. His mentor educated Him in all manner of understanding at the time, which included astronomy, mathematics, history, religion, culture, politics, and more. As was customary at the time, His academic education paralleled His spiritual education. He was taught to read and write using the Torah (the first five books of the Old Testament) and other Jewish holy writ. Evidence of Jesus' appetite to learn and of His advanced knowledge and understanding beyond His years is found in the second chapter of Luke: "...they found him in the temple sitting in the midst of the doctors, both hearing them, and asking them questions. And all that heard him were astonished at his understanding and answers" (Luke 2:46-47).

In modern-day revelation given to Joseph Smith, we are instructed to "...seek...out of the best books words of wisdom; seek learning, even by study and also by faith" and "...study and learn, and become acquainted with all good books, and with languages, tongues, and people" (D&C 88:118; D&C 90:15). Additional revelation tells us that we should study "...things both in heaven and in the earth, and under the earth; things which have been, things which are, things which must shortly come to pass; things which are at home, things which are abroad; the wars and the perplexities of the nations, and the judgments which are on the land; and a knowledge also of countries and of kingdoms" (D&C 88:79).

What you study and learn will make a significant difference in your knowledge, understanding, attitudes, and beliefs. Gaining this depth and breadth of knowledge will allow you to be "...prepared in all things when [the Lord] shall send you...whereunto [He has] called you, and the mission with which [He has] commissioned you" (D&C 88:80). You will be better prepared to understand and communicate more effectively with a wider diversity of people.

Now, because there is so much knowledge to be learned and so many resources for this knowledge, it is imperative you seek out and learn from only uplifting and inspiring sources. Do not waste your valuable time on things that only serve to pollute and destroy your mind. Avoid immoral, violent, or demeaning forms of education and entertainment found in movies, documentaries, television, music, and video games "for the mind through which this filth passes is never the same afterwards" (*Ensign*, May 1986: 45).

PHYSICAL PREPARATION

Jesus was very active as a young boy. During His time, physical activity was necessary for everyone in order to perform even the simplest daily chore. Intense physical activity was an accepted part of everyday life. On several occasions Jesus walked great distances with His family, beginning with His escape to Egypt from King Herod's decree to slay all young boys and continuing annually with long trips from Nazareth to Jerusalem to attend the sacred Jewish festivals. Each trip took Him and His family over dusty and rocky paths, through dry deserts, and over rough mountainous terrain. It was extremely hot during the summer months and extremely cold during the winter months. In part, these intense trips helped Jesus develop great cardiovascular endurance and strong, limber muscles. More importantly, He developed a strong mindset as He endured the discomforts associated with the travels.

As a young, Jewish boy, Jesus began training for a skill that could serve Him well throughout His life. Traditionally, Jewish boys inherited the profession of their father and being raised by a carpenter, Jesus was naturally taught in this trade. Not very many people could endure the physically demanding life of a carpenter. It was a difficult and strenuous profession requiring a great deal of strength and stamina. As such, carpentry was one of the most respected trades at the time.

Jesus dutifully performed this trade as a young man and throughout His adult life until He began His mortal ministry. It was no accident that Jesus was raised by a carpenter. It was God's will to subject His Only Begotten Son to a life of physical hardship in order to prepare Him for His "real" calling. The years of arduous labor endured by Jesus prepared His body for an intense mortal ministry. Jesus traded the callused hands of a carpenter for the callused feet of a street preacher.

From the time Jesus began His mortal ministry, He tirelessly traveled in search of those needing the gospel message and His healing touch. Jesus' area of ministry stretched several miles from Galilee to Jerusalem. The preferred mode of transportation for Jesus was His own two feet. Coincidentally, this is the same approach most missionaries use today. Willingly, missionaries travel the world teaching of Jesus and of the restored gospel while walking among the people just as Jesus did over two-thousand years ago.

The most obvious example demonstrating Jesus'

physical preparation and abilities was during His final days in mortality. Only a strong and well-conditioned Savior could have endured such suffering in the Garden of Gethsemane, the unjust beatings, the torture, being forced to carry His own cross to the location of His crucifixion, and His last breath as a mortal man. Jesus used His well-conditioned body to serve God. He would not have been able to do so without such health and strength. The physical demands He endured during His life was in preparation for what He would undergo during the selfless ordeal we know as the Atonement.

Obviously, you will not be asked or expected to endure the same physical trials and tribulations as the Savior, but missionary work is demanding. It requires good health, physical strength, endurance, and discipline.

How well you feel during your mission and how well you adjust to the environment of your mission is due in large part to how you prepare yourself physically. You are an instrument to the Lord in fulfilling His mission and your body is your instrument in fulfilling your mission. How well your body functions will determine how well the Lord can use you as His instrument. This point is illustrated in the following guideline given to priesthood leaders:

"Disability in the mission field is expensive, embarrassing, and almost always results in detriment to the missionary, his companion, the missionary work, and the church. Any physical weakness or impairments are almost always accentuated by the extensive walking, irregular living conditions, and requirements that accompany missionary living" (*General Handbook of Instructions*, 173).

President Spencer W. Kimball said that serving a mission "...is not an eight- or ten-hour-a-day job. Your whole time, energy, and soul should be turned to this work. It is more than ten or fifteen hours; it is a twenty-four-hour job, at any place that you might happen to be. You need sufficient sleep, not any more. You of course, should eat good wholesome food and have what rest and relaxation are necessary, but the rest of the time belongs to this program to which you have consecrated your life" (Kimball, 575).

The physical preparation for your mission incorporates a variety of factors. It is a multifaceted endeavor involving proper nutrition, sufficient rest, adequate physical exercise, and healthy lifestyle habits. Prior to a mission, conditions are pretty much under your control. You can eat a healthy, well-balanced diet, get plenty of rest, and follow an exercise routine. However, as soon as you leave for your mission, all of this changes. So many unknowns await you. Your diet will no longer be monitored or provided by a loving mother. Your ability to exercise will be severely compromised because of time and equipment constraints. About the only thing that may remain constant is the amount of rest you will get, and perhaps this will even change due to the stress of being in a new environment.

It is important that each of these factors be addressed and properly balanced before leaving on your mission and should continue to be addressed during your mission and throughout your life. If you make these things a priority throughout your mission you will better magnify your divine calling as a representative of the Lord and reach your full potential as a missionary. There is nothing quite as rewarding as fulfilling your potential in every aspect of your life.

As you prepare for your mission, use this book to learn how to eat a well-balanced diet and to prepare and cook meals that provide adequate nutrition. Read and understand the Word of Wisdom (see D&C 89) and follow the do's and the do not's contained therein, which is to eat plenty of vegetables, fresh fruits, and grains while avoiding tobacco, alcohol, coffee, tea, and other harmful or addictive substances. As you do this, you will be blessed as promised at the end of the eighty-ninth section of the Doctrine and Covenants where it reads, "And all saints who remember to keep and do these sayings, walking in obedience to the commandments, shall receive health in their navel and marrow to their bones; And shall find wisdom and great treasures of knowledge, even hidden treasures; And shall run and not be weary, and shall walk and not faint. And I, the Lord, give unto them a promise, that the destroying angel shall pass by them, as the children of Israel, and not slay them" (D&C 89:18-21).

You should follow the counsel of Church leaders as they suggest that, "health preparation [should] begin at least two years in advance of the anticipated missionary service" (*Ensign*, March 2007: 63). Begin an exercise program, such as the one found in this book, and follow it consistently before your mission call comes to establish this daily habit. This can be accomplished by participating in athletic activities or by engaging in other forms of physical exercise like running or lifting weights. Regular physical activity will increase your ability to work and adapt to the rigorous missionary lifestyle as well as the stress that comes along with it. Starting your physical preparation for your mission early and regularly following an exercise program will also lessen the shock of having to exercise each morning while on your mission.

Just as important as physical activity is the principle of rest. Before your mission call comes, you should establish good sleeping patterns. Follow the counsel the Lord has given on the matter: "...cease to sleep longer than is needful; retire to thy bed early, that ye may not be weary; arise early, that your bodies and minds may be invigorated" (D&C 88:124).

In order to have a testimony of the importance to prepare physically for your mission, it is vital to understand the sacred nature of the wonderful gift God has given you – the gift of your physical body and the sacred responsibility you have to care for it.

In the pre-mortal life we understood some vital truths concerning our eternal progression. We knew that our spirits could not reach their full potential without a physical body (see D&C 93:33-34). We knew that our physical bodies would be created in the image of our Heavenly Father. These bodies would be eternal and would be a tabernacle for our spirits. We knew that we would experience a mortal existence, which included pain and pleasure, strength and weakness, health and sickness, self-control and temptations. Despite all of this, or perhaps because of this, we enthusiastically chose to accept the mortal realities of having a physical body.

Satan understands, very clearly, the same eternal truths and principles we were taught in the pre-mortal life concerning our physical bodies. He tries to twist these truths to persuade us down paths contrary to what Heavenly Father desires for us. He does everything in his power to get us to defile, disrespect, and even disregard this beautiful gift God has given us to enjoy. Initially, following one of these paths may feel like freedom, but ultimately it only leads to entrapment and misery. This is one of Satan's ways of rebelling against Father; by getting us to belittle this valuable gift we have been given. Satan persuades us to do this by tempting each person in a different way depending on individual strengths and weaknesses. Some may over-indulge in food, drugs, and other harmful or addictive substances that trap and enslave the user by taking away another precious gift – the gift of agency. Some may disfigure their body with piercings and tattoos, while others seek physical pleasure through immoral behavior. Some may spend too much time on their physical appearance and beauty, while others do not spend enough time on these things. Some people may hate their body, while others worship it.

Each situation is different, but the end result is the same. We start to look at our bodies in a different manner from what our Heavenly Father intended. These types of behaviors cause us to see our bodies as carnal objects – as bodies of flesh and blood only. Instead, we should view our bodies as something much more – as sacred tabernacles that house our spirits.

Jesus was the first to teach that the body is a temple by referring to Himself as a temple (see John 2:19, 21). The apostle Paul later testified to the people of Corinth on the importance of our bodies when he said, "Know ye not that ye are the temple of God, and that the Spirit of God dwelleth in you? If any man defile the temple of God, him shall God destroy; for the temple of God is holy, which temple ye are" (1 Corinthian 3:16-17).

Our bodies are literally temples because they not only house our personal spirits, but they also house the Spirit of God. God honors us by allowing His Spirit to dwell within us so long as we honor Him. This is a great privilege, but with it comes great responsibility. We have been given stewardship over our physical bodies to properly care for them. We must do all in our power to keep our bodies healthy and pure to ensure they are suitable for our spirits and the Spirit of God to dwell within us.

Dr. Kenneth Cooper writes, "[Christians] believe, quite rightly, that the spiritual dimensions of their lives are of supreme importance. But then they proceed to the assumption that their physical bodies are unimportant and may be neglected with impunity. They fail to understand that their spiritual lives – including the values and relationships that they hold so dear - are closely connected with the condition of their bodies. If the body begins to break down, the person may lack the endurance and energy required to serve others, stay in a good mood, or even spend extended periods in prayer" (Cooper, 24-25). If we do not keep our bodies in optimal health, then we become incapable of serving God to the best of our abilities.

The care of our physical body is a spiritual obligation. There is a very close and real relationship between our physical health and our spiritual development. The healthier the body, the greater capacity it has to obey; the weaker the body, the more it demands. As the desires of the flesh grow, the influence of the spirit fades. If the body is not functioning correctly as it was designed, then it becomes much more difficult for the spirit to rule over it.

As you properly care for your body, it will function more effectively and efficiently. The fact that God's Spirit is within you should be reason enough to keep your body healthy and fit. However, if this is not enough to motivate you, consider the following reasons: You will be able to serve more powerfully bringing joy to you and to those you serve. You will be a more influential example. It takes a lot of energy, stamina, and strength to be a good example. You will have more confidence in yourself. As you keep your body healthy, you will feel good and, in turn, you will have a better attitude about your own life and the lives of others. You will be more kind, loving, and patient. Overall, you will be a more powerful and effective missionary, more capable of serving to the best of your ability. President David O. McKay said, "The healthy man, who takes care of his physical being, has strength and vitality; his temple is a fit place for his spirit to reside... It is necessary, therefore, to care for our physical bodies, and observe the laws of physical health and happiness" (*Improvement Era*, April 1952: 221). Fortunately, this book will address each of the physical factors in greater detail in order to help you prepare and serve a physically healthy mission.

SPIRITUAL PREPARATION

Two significant events recorded in scriptures stand out in regard to Jesus' spiritual preparation. One prepared Him for His mortal ministry while the other prepared Him for His eternal ministry.

Immediately following His baptism, Jesus was led by the Spirit into the wilderness of Judea. There, He received spiritual guidance, strength, and instruction from Heavenly Father and other heavenly beings preparing Him further for His ministry (see Matthew 4:1-2; Mark 1:12-13; Luke 4:1-2). Without concern for food or water and in an isolated environment, Jesus had the opportunity to fully devote His time, energy, and attention to communing with Heavenly Father to receive eternal knowledge from on high. This experience taught Him how to subject the will of His body to the will of His spirit, furthering His ability to withstand temptations and other physical trials that would come.

After forty days and nights Jesus came out of His wilderness sanctuary spiritually strong but physically weak. Surely, one of His first priorities was to quench His thirst and satisfy His hunger pangs. However, this would have to wait as He was quickly confronted by the adversary. Satan proceeded to tempt Jesus with temptations that appeal to the natural appetites of all mankind. He tempted Jesus by saying, "If thou be the Son of God, command that these stones be made bread" (Matthew 4:3). A simple taunting by Satan to command a stone to turn into bread would have been an easy task for Jesus. All He had to do was usurp His ability to control the elements and command a few stones to be made bread. Jesus effortlessly thwarted the temptation when He said, "It is written, Man shall not live by bread alone, but by every word that proceedeth out of the mouth of God" (Matthew 4:4).

The response Jesus gave refers to the very statement Moses made to the Israelites concerning the manna they were blessed to receive during their forty years in the wilderness (see Deuteronomy 8:3). Bruce R. McConkie commented, "Even as Israel relied upon Jehovah for their daily bread, lest they die physically, so they must rely upon him for the word of God, which is spiritual bread, lest they die spiritually. Neither temporal nor spiritual bread, standing alone, will suffice; man must eat of both to live; and in the eternal sense, the word of God, which is the bread from heaven in the full sense, is the more important. Those who make the search for earthly bread their chief concern lose sight of eternal values, fail to feed their spirits, die spiritually, and lose their souls... [Jesus], as the Son of God, chooses the bread from heaven and will find earthly food when his circumstances permit. He is master over the flesh; his appetites will be kept within the bounds set by divine standards" (McConkie, *Mortal Messiah*, 413). Triumphantly, Jesus dismissed the other two attempts to ensnare Him and then casually dismissed Satan without consequence.

This experience parallels Jesus' most spiritually and physically demanding task of all – the Atonement. As the scriptures record, the final night of His mortal ministry was spent in preparation, communing with God just as He had begun His ministry in the wilderness three years before. Ironically, Jesus prepared for such a bright ministry in a dreary wilderness and prepared for such a dreary ending to His mortal ministry in a beautiful garden. The wilderness was a rough environment weakening Him physically, but strengthening Him spiritually. The Garden of Gethsemane was a peaceful place where He would be weakened physically and tested spiritually. In both situations Jesus was afforded the quiet time needed to reflect and gain strength from on high.

Just as Jesus prepared spiritually long before His ministry began, your spiritual preparation should begin long before you begin your mission. Aside from the brief instruction given at the Missionary Training Center, you receive relatively little specific and formal training for your mission. The majority of your spiritual preparation for your mission will come from your own personal study of the gospel, teachings from your parents, attending church meetings, and attending seminary and/or institute. In addition, there are countless books and other resources available to assist you in your spiritual preparation.

The details of preparing spiritually for your mission are beyond the scope of this book. However, you will know that you are spiritually prepared to serve the Lord on a mission when you have developed the following desires:

- A desire to pray regularly and commune with Heavenly Father

- A desire to study the scriptures daily and apply the principles in your life

- A desire to share your testimony of the Gospel of Jesus Christ

- A desire to honor and respect your priesthood

- A desire to serve others with a joyful heart

- A desire to be humble

- A desire to keep your life clean, in thoughts and actions

- A desire to be obedient to the commandments

SOCIAL PREPARATION

Growing up as a carpenter, Jesus was only as successful as His skills allowed. The skills to ensure His success were not just limited to His ability to shape wood into useful, everyday items. No matter how exquisite His works of craftsmanship were, no one could appreciate them unless Jesus possessed the ability to sell His creations. Jesus would have learned people skills and would have grown in confidence in His ability to communicate with others as He described the features and benefits of each product or as He listened and understood a customer who came to Him for a custom-made piece. He became well-liked and respected as He honestly and fairly dealt with those whom He did business. His confidence and ability to communicate demanded the respect of others. This carried over into His ministry as He taught the gospel and performed many miracles. His love and charisma won over many disciples to His worthy cause.

A mission requires this same confidence and ability to communicate with others. It requires faith in oneself and in understanding your divine nature as a literal child of God. Become the type of person others want to be around and associate with. By following these guidelines you will become that person:

- Learn to communicate with others. Be a good listener. Remember you have two ears and only one mouth. This means you should listen twice as much as you speak. Only after listening should you express your thoughts in an honest and sincere manner.

- Learn to get along with others. Focus on what you have in common with others and on their good qualities. Do not let differences stand in the way of your relationships. Become genuinely interested in others and in their interests and desires. More than anything else, this will help you get along with your companions and other missionaries with whom you serve.

- Learn to be gracious and well-mannered. Behave appropriately in every situation observing good manners and speaking politely and with respect to others and about others.

- Learn to lead and to follow. Be grateful for the opportunities you have to lead, but even more grateful for the opportunities you will have to follow. Show respect for your leaders because someday you may be in their position and you will want the same respect shown to you.

- Learn to love. Follow the example of Christ and develop charity as He has encouraged us. This will be one of the most valuable attributes you can possess.

During your time as a missionary you will develop some of the most lasting friendships and relationships of your life. You will meet missionaries, members, and investigators who will touch your life in ways no one else can and you will touch their lives in a similar manner. These friendships will have an everlasting effect on you and your life. Be prepared socially so you can make the most of your friendships and relationships.

Jesus was the embodiment of perfection. He showed us how to live, love, teach, forgive, and to be good stewards. He healed the sick, raised the dead, and conquered physical and spiritual death for everyone. Clearly, Jesus lived a well-balanced, healthy lifestyle and was the perfect example in all aspects of life.

Just like Jesus, everyone has mental, physical,

spiritual, and social needs that must be developed and nurtured continuously in order to stay well-balanced and in harmony with our Heavenly Father and the teachings of the gospel. If we fail to develop in any of these areas, then it will eventually suffer and become a burden. The tragedy is that if one area falls out of balance or is neglected, every other area will suffer. First Corinthians 12:26 reads, "And whether one member suffer, all the members suffer with it."

Make the commitment now to prepare yourself in each of these four areas and continue that preparation throughout your mission and your life. Enjoy the preparation process. It is a continual process, but one that will increase your ability to perform to your fullest potential as a missionary.

All of your physical and spiritual preparations will soon be realized once you get to the Missionary Training Center. However, all this preparation may be in vain unless you have packed a few necessary items in order to take full advantage of it. The next chapter will help you know what to bring in order to maintain your physical and spiritual health while on your mission.

PACKING WITH FITNESS IN MIND

Entering the mission field without the right stuff is almost as disastrous as entering the mission field without correct knowledge of the gospel. A lack of "tools" makes your job as a missionary more difficult to completely focus on serving the Lord. Since you will be gone for 18 or 24 months, you will need to plan carefully what to bring on your mission and what to leave at home.

When you receive your mission call it will be accompanied with a packet of information. Included with this information are the official church guidelines on what you should pack for your mission. This list will include everything from clothing to toiletries. Be sure to include all of the items it suggests. Shortly after you receive your mission call, another letter and packet should arrive from the mission president of your mission. In this letter he will outline specifics about the culture and climate of your appointed mission and will usually indicate anything else you should pack in addition to the list you previously received. Heed his counsel because, as the mission president, he knows what the specific needs are for your particular mission.

It can be tedious and even frustrating when you are trying to find all of the essential items you will need to pack for your mission. This can be especially difficult if you don't know where to look or what to look for in terms of quality and material selection. Most of the dress clothes found at regular department stores are not made to withstand the constant wear and tear that rigorous mission life demands. Unfortunately, a lot of missionaries will buy lesser-quality items in an effort to save money only to find out the hard way when their pants or shirts wear-out after only a few short months in the mission field.

Fortunately, there is a company that understands these issues and provides the products to overcome them. Missionary Mall is the "one-stop-shop" where you can get everything you need from the official mission list at the best prices around. Since most of the products they provide are specifically made for missionaries they meet the highest standards of quality and are guaranteed for two years to withstand the rigors of mission life. Missionary Mall stands behind this promise by being the only missionary supplier who will replace any item for free if it wears out, rips, tears, breaks, falls apart, etc. during the two years following its purchase.

Since 1997 they've proudly assisted over half the missionary population with a friendly and knowledgeable staff of experts. Comprised only of returned missionaries, the staff will educate you throughout the entire purchasing process. Stop by any of their store locations or visit them online at www.missionarymall.org for an easy and cost-effective way to gear up for "the greatest work in all the world."

In addition to packing all the necessary items from the official church guidelines, here are some additional items and tips you may want to consider when packing for your mission.

FOCUS ON TRAVELING LIGHT

Most missionaries have a tendency to over-pack, bringing too much into the mission field. All too often, a missionary begins his mission with several suitcases or bags stuffed beyond their capacity. After the first month or so the missionary realizes he has not used any of the extra things he packed. As a result, he ends up making a trip to the local post office to send a box or two of the unused items home, costing him and his family unnecessary time and expensive shipping charges.

By planning ahead and packing only the things you will need, you can keep your luggage as light and as manageable as possible while you travel to and from your mission and transfer to various areas within your mission. The most important thing is to choose a set of luggage that is lightweight for ease of travel yet durable enough to withstand the constant handling during the course of your mission. The luggage you pick should include retractable handles, wide, padded shoulder straps, multiple grab handles for ease of maneuvering in any situation, partially recessed wheels, reinforced stitching around the zippers, pockets, and handles, and multiple layers of fabric or extra reinforcement on the corners and edges for durability.

Include with your luggage a backpack with a built-in pouch or sleeve to hold a water reservoir so you can more easily meet all of your hydration needs. This is perhaps the simplest and most convenient way to re-hydrate during your mission. This pack should be big enough to accommodate your scriptures, teaching materials, snacks, and anything else you might need to bring along with you during a typical day in the mission field.

Use travel-size containers for shampoo, lotion, toothpaste, mouthwash, deodorant, and other toiletries. Put these small containers into re-sealable plastic bags to keep their contents from getting all over your clothes and the inside of your luggage if they spill or leak. There is nothing worse than arriving in your mission or in a new area to find all of your white shirts need to be washed before you can wear them because they have shampoo all over them. Wearing the same shirt until the next P-day will not be a pleasant experience for you or your companion!

Limit the number of shoes you pack. They are usually the heaviest things you will pack and they take up a lot of room. You will only need to pack one good pair of comfortable, lightweight, and sturdy athletic shoes. A good, quality pair should last you the entire duration of your mission. You will not be using them often enough to wear them out during 18 or 24 months. The athletic shoes will be used during your daily exercise time as well as your preparation day activities, so choose a pair that will accommodate the type of activities you anticipate participating in the most, whether it is running, playing basketball, or whatever. The best solution if you expect to take part in a variety of activities might be to buy a pair of cross-trainers. This type of athletic shoe can safely and comfortably be used for almost any activity.

Bring only two pairs of dress shoes. Be very specific with the type of dress shoes you buy. Remember, you will wear these shoes nearly every day of your mission. They need to look like dress shoes, but feel more like athletic shoes and meet the requirements set forth by your mission president. No matter where you serve, you will do a great deal of walking and standing on your mission and you do not want to experience any more blisters or in-grown toenails than are likely to occur. Most dress shoes, although nice looking, are not always comfortable to wear and are designed to be worn for only a few hours at a time with limited walking. Because of this, you should consider buying dress shoes that have athletic or rubber soles, are made with soft leather, and are lightweight. Also, make sure they are sturdy and comfortable, providing good ankle support with solid arches to help maintain balance while protecting your feet.

PACK ITEMS THAT SERVE MULTIPLE FUNCTIONS

The obvious example of this is to pack socks that are dark athletic socks instead of packing thin dress socks that give little support and wear-out quickly. Dark-colored athletic socks will last longer, are more comfortable, more supportive, can be worn while exercising or tracting, and are designed to wick moisture away more effectively.

Buy socks with the same color and pattern. Several black or dark, navy blue socks are ideal colors. Doing this will always allow you to have a matching pair in case you lose one in the laundry or one gets a hole worn in it. Simply pair the odd sock up with another one. By doing this, you will avoid any embarrassing moments of wearing two mismatched socks during an important meeting or discussion.

For a professional look, make sure your dress pants and suits all match your socks, belts, and shoes. For example, black shoes, black socks, and a black belt. Black is a good color choice for these items, because black will almost always go with any other color of clothing. As a missionary there is not a lot of room for variety in styles and fashion choices. Remember, you are a representative of the Lord, not yourself. About the only variety in your daily wardrobe will come in your necktie selection. Always choose ties that are conservative in color, width, and design, with no pictures or bright colors that may be distracting from the Gospel message.

Before leaving home for your mission, give your parents a list of your shoe, shirt, suit, and pant sizes for the different styles and brands of clothing you will be wearing. This will save you and your parents a lot of time, effort, and money by getting it right the first time, instead of finding the right fit through trial and error. Make sure to update your parents with your most current sizes as your body may grow and change throughout your mission.

PACK APPROPRIATE CLOTHES FOR PHYSICAL ACTIVITY

In addition to the recommended guidelines for the clothes you should pack, consider bringing an extra set or two of gym clothes. You will need two to three sets so when one set is soiled, waiting to be cleaned, you will still have another set or two to use. This is not only a good idea for convenience, but also for cleanliness and hygiene. It is not good to wear soiled clothing again and again without washing them. Bacteria and other microorganisms can begin to grow on the clothing which may cause health concerns.

Pack two or three loose-fitting or stretchable, lightweight t-shirts and shorts that allow perspiration to evaporate quickly. Include a couple pair of athletic socks that can also wick moisture away quickly. This type of clothing is easy to rinse out and dries quickly, which is a plus when laundry facilities are hard to come by or when you are limited to washing once each week. Another piece of exercise clothing you should bring is a pair of sweats - a sweatshirt and sweatpants. This will especially be helpful in colder climates.

Make sure the gym clothes you bring are modest. They should always cover your garments, regardless of whether you wear your garments or not during exercise. Also be sure to pack two to three pair of appropriate undergarments for physical activities - supportive jock straps or briefs for elders and sports bras for sisters.

A side note about your temple garments and exercise: You should always wear your garments when performing exercise and most other physical activities. There may be some exceptions to this practice, but check with your mission president beforehand. Following any exercise or physical activity and after you have showered, put on a clean, fresh pair of garments and, respectfully, place the soiled pair of garments in the appropriate place to be laundered later.

PACK TO ACCOMMODATE YOUR FITNESS NEEDS

To consistently follow an exercise program while on your mission, you need determination, realistic expectations, and a willingness to adapt. Having a positive attitude and mindset however, will only get you so far. You also need the right "tools" to ensure your success. Unfortunately, missionary apartments do not double as fitness centers and access to fitness centers are rare and perhaps even against mission rules. This presents a unique dilemma since you are expected to exercise each morning on your mission.

Fortunately, daily exercise can effectively be achieved while serving your mission without the need to go to a local fitness center or having to buy and pack expensive and bulky equipment. All you need are a few well-selected items along with your own bodyweight to guarantee an excellent workout each day. Each piece of exercise equipment you pack must meet certain specifications. Each must be small and compact, inexpensive and lightweight, quick and easy to set-up and use, versatile, portable, and convenient.

Following is a list of the items meeting all of the above guidelines you need to turn your missionary apartment and the surrounding area into a Missionary Fitness gym.

Bodyweight

The first piece of equipment is the cheapest and most convenient because everyone already has it – it is your own body. As long as gravity exists, the weight of your body can provide an effective workout that rivals any resistance-training routine using iron weights. Your body serves as the best piece of equipment because it is the right size, the right weight, it's portable, travels easily, and is always available.

A major misconception people have about bodyweight exercises is that they can only build muscular endurance and bodyweight exercises alone are not capable of increasing or maintaining any significant level of muscular strength or muscle mass. However, by simply redistributing the body between the limbs, manipulating the range of motion, performing the exercise in an unstable environment, varying the leverage, or by minimizing momentum, it becomes possible to increase muscular strength, size, and endurance.

The best example of this is elite-level gymnasts. They have very lean, well-toned, and powerful physiques. They train and build their strength and physiques primarily from bodyweight exercises alone, day-in and day-out. In the same way gymnasts develop their muscular strength, definition, and mass, you too can develop great results by following an exercise program utilizing bodyweight exercises as the foundation, supplemented with exercises using the following equipment.

Exercise Tubing and Bands

The fitness industry has spent millions of dollars to design and build costly machines that essentially do what inexpensive elastic tubing and bands can do just as well, and in some cases, better. The great thing about exercise tubing and bands is their ability to provide variable levels of resistance in all three planes of movement and throughout the entire range of motion. Resistance for any exercise can be easily controlled by using tubing or bands of different thicknesses, by stretching them out to various lengths, or a combination of both. In this way they also require the user to maintain control and stability throughout the movement.

Exercise tubing or bands are probably the single most useful resistance-training equipment, besides your own bodyweight, that you can bring with you on your mission. They can provide you with a great workout, are extremely light and portable, can be used almost anywhere, are inexpensive, and are an easy way for any missionary, no matter what level of exercise experience you have, to develop functional strength and general conditioning.

A note of caution: Exercise tubing and bands can be very dangerous and can cause serious injury when not used properly. Use exercise tubing and bands according to the manufacturer's recommended guidelines. Do not use them in any manner that may cause them to snap towards you, your vital body parts; including your head, face, and eyes, or anyone else and their vital body parts. Although tempting, exercise tubing and bands are not toys and should never be used as such.

Other Forms of Resistance

Exercise tubing and bands will be your best form of resistance besides your own bodyweight while on your mission. However, additional forms of resistance can be used if they become available. Bags, backpacks, jugs, containers, paint cans, and buckets all have their own built-in handles or straps and can be filled with water, sand, cement, books, or any other heavy objects to increase resistance. These forms of resistance are not as compact or as portable, but are relatively inexpensive and can easily be found in almost any area you serve.

Exercise Ball

Exercise balls are great because they require the body to recruit small, stabilizing muscles in order to stay balanced and on top of the ball. This allows you to develop stability, balance, and coordination, especially in the core area, while working on muscular strength, size, or endurance. They help train the muscles to work in unison, mimicking real-world movements. Utilizing this piece of equipment adds more variety to any exercise program because of the limitless variety of exercises that can be performed with them.

If you are not able to use an exercise ball, then some alternatives can be used. Essentially, you can use anything that is solid enough to hold your bodyweight. Whatever it is, it should be between 12 and 18-inches wide and long enough to support your body, shoulders, neck, and head. It should raise your body above the floor by several inches so when performing exercises, your arms can move freely without your elbows touching the ground.

Some alternative items may include a piano bench, a park bench, two chairs put together, a few pillows or couch cushions stacked on top of each other, a sturdy coffee table, a wood plank with two or three phone books under each end to raise the board to the desired height (create an incline or decline bench by adding more phone books to one side or the other), or the phone books alone will also work.

Jump Rope

Jump ropes provide excellent energy system workouts. You can jump rope just about anywhere – in your apartment, on the front porch, on the sidewalk, in the grass, etc. Just make sure there is enough clearance above your head if you are inside so you do not hit the ceiling or any light fixtures.

The best type of jump rope is a "speed rope," a thin, lightweight rope made of soft plastic. Make sure to choose a jump rope that is either adjustable or is already set at the right length for your height. A jump rope that is too short will catch your feet as it goes around and one that is too long will be difficult to get around without losing speed and momentum. To find the right length for your jump rope, stand on the center of the rope with your feet together and pull the handles towards your shoulders. The handles of the jump rope should be within a few inches of your armpits.

Exercise Straps

Exercise straps are made out of nylon webbing with adjustable handles and can be secured to any solid overhead bar or anchored behind the top of any sturdy, closed door. The suspended design of the exercise strap allows you to increase or decrease the resistance of hundreds of exercises, including a variety of pull-ups, push-ups, and dips by varying the angle of your body in relation to the strap.

Each of the above-mentioned items can be found at any sporting goods store or most discount shopping centers. To learn more about how to utilize these pieces of exercise equipment in your daily exercise program a companion guide to this book has been compiled and is titled: *Additional Exercises for Missionary Fitness*. It is available at www.missionaryfitness.com.

Exercise and Nutrition Journal

It is tough enough trying to remember your daily schedule with all of your many appointments and meetings, let alone your exercise and nutrition program. In the same way you have a planner to keep track of your daily schedule of appointments and meetings; you should also keep a planner of sorts for your exercise and nutrition information. By documenting and keeping a detailed record of your exercise and nutrition program, you will be more successful in meeting your health needs and fitness goals.

Keeping records of your workouts and meals in an exercise and nutrition journal allow you to chart vital information. Regularly evaluating and accurately tracking this information can be a valuable source of accountability and motivation. Keeping such a record allows for daily self-analysis where you can recognize progress, thus building confidence in the process, or you can identify reasons in failing to progress. You can look back and see what the contributing factors or patterns were to your success or demise and make the necessary adjustments and changes before it is too late.

You can create your own exercise and nutrition journal by documenting the important elements of your workout and diet in your weekly planner or you can visit www.missionaryfitness.com to download and print a free copy of the companion journal to this book titled: *Missionary Fitness Journal*.

With all the necessary items packed and ready to go, you are well on your way to the start of a rewarding and fulfilling journey as a servant of the Lord. The first stop on your journey is one you will never forget! It is the Missionary Training Center.

THE MTC EXPERIENCE

The first stop on your mission as a newly called missionary is the Missionary Training Center. Depending on what mission you are called to will determine which of the several Missionary Training Centers you will attend. Regardless of which Missionary Training Center you go to, you will still participate in the same basic experience as every other missionary. They all follow the same daily schedule and training curriculum, use the same teaching materials and systems, and have the same purpose.

The Missionary Training Center or MTC as it is commonly referred to, will be your new home for the next three, eight, or twelve weeks, depending on the specific language you may need to learn. It will prove to be a very unique and extremely spiritual experience designed to help you understand your assignment as a missionary, to help you develop the necessary skills to be a successful missionary, and to prepare you in all aspects of missionary service.

FIRST DAY

Upon arriving at the MTC, you will first check in and be issued a name tag with your new title. Next, you will be instructed to put your luggage in a holding room and attend an orientation meeting with your family if they made the trip with you. Family members who are able to come will be allowed to sit next to you for the last time until you return home after your mission. During this meeting the MTC president and his wife will spend a few moments welcoming you and assuring your family that you are in good hands. Then you will watch a video presentation showing you and your family what to expect during your stay at the MTC.

After only about 30 minutes, the meeting comes to an end and it is time to say good-bye to your family. Following some hugs, kisses, and tears exchanged between you and your family, they are ushered out one side of the room and you are ushered out the other side of the room to begin the rest of your mission.

At the next stop in another area of the MTC, you will receive an information packet, which includes your daily schedule, companion's name, residence hall and district assignment, room number and key, branch president's information, a debit card, and your valuable mailbox number. Volunteers will be on hand to answer any questions you might have and to usher you through the induction process. The next couple of hours will consist of filling out paperwork, reporting any health or dietary issues, receiving any immunizations you may need, and picking up all the necessary study materials and workbooks at the MTC bookstore.

After retrieving your luggage from the holding room, you will then find your dorm room where you will begin to unpack and meet your new companion and other members of your district. From this time forward, you will be with this companion while at the MTC. You will both be a source of strength, support, and protection for each other. You may immediately find that you and your companion get along well. Others may have to spend a little more time developing their relationship. Together, you and your companion will be expected to keep a very tight schedule.

The daily schedule from your information packet will indicate when and where you and your companion should be during your entire stay at the MTC. The schedule at the MTC has been carefully designed through study, observation, prayer, and inspiration to properly balance all the essential aspects of effectively preparing a missionary for mission service. This carefully planned schedule will account for blocks of time for classroom instruction, meals, service assignments, laundry, personal time, gym time, and temple attendance. Take advantage of the MTC experience and all that it has to offer, exactly as it is offered. You will not get another opportunity to experience it again, not even in the mission field.

The next thing on the schedule for your first day is another more detailed, orientation explaining the organization of the MTC and the services available to you. Dinner is next followed by another meeting where you will meet your branch presidency. Your branch president will preside over Sunday meetings and conduct personal interviews with you during your time there. At the end of an exhausting first day, having received a lot of information and meeting several new people, you will be ready to go to sleep when its time for the lights to go out.

THE TRAINING BEGINS

The next day and every other day during your stay at the MTC will typically begin at 6:00 a.m. Each day includes personal and companionship study time, breakfast, classroom instruction, lunch, classroom instruction, dinner, more classroom instruction, and then it is off to bed at 10:30 p.m. for another well-deserved rest before starting it all over again.

You will be given three meals a day while at the MTC. There will be plenty of food to choose from, but be cautious and make wise choices with your food selection, because with all of the sitting and studying you will do and with so much variety of food to choose from at each and every meal, this presents a potentially bad situation. Many unsuspecting missionaries have added extra weight during their brief stay at the MTC because of a combination of sitting around more than they are used to and having access to an almost endless supply of food. This is not a good way to begin a successful mission! If you are not careful, it may set the mood for the rest of your mission. Be sure to read and follow the suggestions on nutrition and diet found later in this book.

During your time at the MTC, your many classes and trainings will focus around four basic areas: personal development, gospel study, missionary skills and Christ-like attributes, and language and culture.

Personal development classes center on teaching you the proper way to dress and groom, proper etiquette, the importance of health and hygiene, nutrition and physical exercise, safety, money management, and communication skills.

Gospel study includes time for personal scripture study, Sabbath Day worship service, a weekly session at the temple, and a weekly devotional where you will get to listen to prophets, apostles, and other general authorities speak.

In missionary skills and Christ-like attribute classes you will learn how to find and teach people, how to teach by the spirit, and how to present the gospel message in a way that each individual you teach can understand and receive a testimony for themselves.

In language and culture classes, you will be taught by teachers who are from the country in which you will be serving, or who have recently returned home from a mission in that country. They will teach you about the country and the people, the customs and traditions, and the food and cuisine so it is not such a shock when you arrive. They may even show you photographs of what the place looks like or they may bring you food and other treats from that area to try. They will do their best to help you understand your mission so you can adapt to your new surroundings as quickly as possible upon arriving. They will also help you develop your language skills in a way that you will feel more confident in your ability to carry on a basic conversation upon arriving in your mission.

Of course, each day at the MTC is not all eating and sitting in classrooms, although this is how it will feel at times! During each day you will also have the opportunity to take a break from your academic and spiritual studies and give your mind a rest by participating in physical exercise. You will have about 50 minutes to exercise each day, five days per week. During this time you will be able to participate in several different forms of physical activities including basketball, volleyball, running, lifting weights, and more.

Exercising at the MTC will prove to be very beneficial for you because of the long hours sitting in the cafeteria and the classrooms. Your mouth and mind will get plenty of exercise but if you do not give your physical body sufficient attention to balance all of this out, you run the risk of developing unhealthy habits, or worse, burning-out before you even arrive in your assigned mission. These unhealthy habits, unless corrected, may lead to sickness or disability in the mission field, hindering the missionary work in your area.

Take advantage of the time you are given for physical activity and exercise at the MTC. You will find that some missionaries will spend this time catching up on sleep, writing letters to loved ones, spending extra time studying, or just wasting the time away in other pursuits. There will be sufficient time during the day and throughout each week to take care of all your other needs and desires as long as you closely follow the daily schedule as it has been given to you.

By participating in regular physical activity at the MTC your ability to comprehend and retain what you learn in the classrooms will increase. In addition, you will have more energy to sustain you throughout the long days.

PREPARATION TIME

Just like in the mission field, each week at the MTC, you will have preparation time to take care of any personal or practical matters. This time will give you a chance to rest and relax a little and take a break from the rigorous and sometimes demanding routine. You will have the opportunity to go to the temple, do laundry, write letters, go shopping at the bookstore, get a haircut, participate in one of many recreational activities, or go to the gym for some extra physical activity and exercise. You will learn in a later chapter how important preparation time is to the success of your mission.

Start your mission off right and take advantage of the MTC experience. Although, it will be physically, mentally, emotionally, and spiritually demanding, it will also be one of the highlights of your entire mission. As you work hard and are obedient, the Lord will bless you with an increase of His Spirit and you will be fully prepared when your time at the MTC comes to an end.

SECTION II:

COMMITTING TO
MISSIONARY
FITNESS

NOURISHING YOUR BODY

I n order to start and drive a car, it must have a sufficient amount of gasoline in it. Similar to fueling a car, your body needs fuel for energy and for maintaining normal physiological functions. This fuel comes from the nutrients in the food and fluid you eat and drink. What you eat influences how you look, feel, sleep, and ultimately, how you perform as a missionary. To look good, feel energized, rest sufficiently, and perform optimally you need to eat well, which means fueling or nourishing your body with a healthy variety of foods consistently throughout the day.

Besides giving you energy and making you look and feel good, eating healthy also helps prevent the number one inhibitor to missionary work in the mission field – illness. Without proper nutrition, your service as a missionary will suffer and you will be limited in your ability to serve. A sick missionary is restricted to the apartment all day, severely hindering the work in that area.

Unfortunately, mission life is not the ideal situation for healthy eating. Living on a limited budget, eating at fast-food restaurants on a regular basis, snacking on junk-food between appointments, and having a limited selection of foods to choose from can be disastrous to your health. Sadly, in some extreme cases, there have been missionaries who have returned home looking like they spent the better part of their mission at an "all-you-can-eat" buffet instead of preaching the gospel. Do not let this happen to you!

Mainstream media would have you believe that eating healthy is difficult, expensive, time-consuming, complex, and the only way to achieve it is to follow the latest fad diet. In reality, all you really need is some commonsense, a basic understanding of nutrition, and some simple, proven strategies that are easy to follow.

This chapter is not intended to be a review of fundamental nutrition principles. Such a discussion is beyond the scope of a single chapter. Hopefully, you have already acquired a basic understanding of nutrition from a high school or college health course. If not, you can find several nutrition books at your local library to help you gain this knowledge prior to leaving for your mission. With this understanding, you can more effectively implement the information in this chapter. This chapter is, however, intended to provide you with some simple, no-nonsense strategies based on proven scientific principles that will help you decide what to eat and when to eat while serving your mission.

PLAN AND PREPARE YOUR MEALS

The hardest part about following a healthy diet is developing a plan and being prepared. Without proper planning many missionaries will skip meals, graze on high-calorie, low-nutrient foods, and try to make-up for their unsatisfied appetite at night with quick and convenient, unhealthy alternatives. The first thing you must do to avoid this is to plan out each and every meal. An easy way to do this is to take time every preparation day to write out a menu for the coming week. Then go shopping for the groceries you will need based on that menu. Finally, after returning home from shopping, do the preliminary preparations on the food you just bought for each of the meals in your weekly menu.

Start the weekly menu planning by writing down seven different breakfast meals, seven different lunch meals, and seven different dinner meals. You might not need to plan every lunch and dinner meal depending on your area and the number of meal appointments you have in that particular area, so adjust accordingly. Be sure to plan for two or three healthy snacks or "mini-meals" throughout the day. Typically, each of these "mini-meals" will fall between each of the main meals.

After the menu for each meal and "mini-meal" is planned, add up exactly what food and how much of it you will need for the next seven days. Then make a list of the groceries needed for each of the meals. Initially, this step might take an hour or so, but after you have established the first week's meal-plan, and with some practice, each weekly meal-plan after should be much quicker and easier because only a few things will change from week to week. Eventually this step will only take a few minutes.

Now that the meal-plan for the entire week is complete you need to go shopping for the groceries. Just like planning the meals, this step may take an hour or so in the beginning, however, with practice you should be able to complete all of the grocery shopping within thirty-minutes because you will learn exactly what you need and where it is in the store.

After you get back home, you will want to do the preliminary food preparation for all of the meals. This includes cooking the meat, rice, beans, and pasta; chopping and slicing the fruits and vegetables; and measuring out all of the yogurt and cottage cheese for each meal. Now, place each item in its own air-tight, plastic container and store the prepared food in the freezer or refrigerator so it is ready each day, regardless of what comes up in your schedule. Finally, when preparing breakfast each morning, perform the final food preparation for every meal you will need to take along with you as you perform your daily missionary labors. Store each food item in plastic bags or air-tight containers and place them in a small, portable cooler that you can keep with you or carry in your backpack. If your backpack has a water reservoir, the cool water will help insulate the food and keep it fresh all day. If, during the day, you will be returning to your apartment and have sufficient time to prepare the meal, then simply make the final meal preparations at that time in your apartment.

If you are in a mission where local members prepare meals for you, let that person know about your meal-plans and give them your grocery list so they can do the shopping and food preparation accordingly.

SPECIAL CONSIDERATIONS

Transferring into a new area: When transferring into a new area, plan ahead and be prepared by bringing some bottled water, sliced vegetables, fresh fruits, a variety of nuts and seeds, and any other portable, non-perishable food items to eat on the trip. As soon as possible after arriving in your new area go shopping for only the necessary foods to hold you over until your next preparation day. If you do not do this, you will be at the mercy of whatever food is left behind in the cupboards and fridge of your new apartment. This increases your risk of falling victim to bad eating habits. A risk you do not want to take!

Eating out: Eating out is a part of everyday life, and it is certainly part of mission life. Most missionaries will eat out several times a week for obvious reasons. Fast food and other convenient restaurants can be the answer to your prayers when you are on the go between appointments and meetings. But keep in mind, the most nutritious and cost-effective meals will be the ones you prepare yourself. Eating out can be expensive, is typically less healthy, and consumes a lot of valuable time. Therefore, avoid eating out as much as possible. However, there will be times when it is necessary, convenient, or even pleasurable to eat out. At such times, be sure to adhere to the following guidelines:

The serving sizes most restaurants serve are typically much larger than needed. They are generally sufficient for two people or for two meals. Do not feel like you must eat everything on your plate. Split the meal with your companion, plan to take half of it home with you to eat at a later meal, or order an appetizer portion to limit the meal to a healthier quantity.

Look for items on the menu that are grilled, baked, poached, steamed, or broiled and avoid fried foods. Always request the dressings and sauces be served on the side so you can control the amount you eat. Add vegetable side-dishes to your meals and ask that your vegetables be prepared with olive or canola oil instead of butter, shortening, or margarine when they are cooked. Choose vegetable-based soups rather than cream-based soups, request whole-grain bread rather than white bread, and choose to eat fresh fruit for dessert.

Do not think you are limited to the choices on the menu. You do not necessarily need to order what is on the menu. Be aware that most restaurants are happy to accommodate you by making changes and substitutions to your specifications even if it is not on their menu. Feel free to adapt current meals on the menu or custom-order what you want even if it is not on the menu.

Do an internet search of restaurants and other eating establishments in your mission before arriving. In each area of your mission, compile a list of about four restaurants that you know will provide a menu that can match your healthy diet. Two of the restaurants should be fast-food places, and two should be sit-down style restaurants. Visit each restaurant's website, view their menus online, and print them out or have them send you a hard copy. By doing this, you will know exactly how to alter certain meals in order to meet your nutritional needs. Next time everyone is trying to decide which restaurant to go to after a district meeting or zone conference, you can volunteer one of your four choices.

When you do find yourself eating out, take advantage of the valuable opportunity to share the gospel with the people who are also eating out!

Dinner appointments with members: Meals are a great time for members to get to know the missionaries in the area. Depending on your mission you might have the opportunity to eat meals with members on a regular basis. This is a convenient luxury that presents a whole new set of circumstances that you must effectively manage in order to maintain a healthy diet. At first it may seem that these appointments are completely out of your control. However, if you follow these guidelines when eating at members' homes, you will be able to maintain a healthy diet and serve a more productive mission:

Limit your eating appointments with members to only three meals per week. This saves time, lessens the burden for members, and helps keep you healthy. Call each member who has scheduled a meal with you in advance to inform them of your food restrictions, allergies, or other dietary concerns you or your companion may have. When doing this, be sensitive and understanding of the member's financial means and ability to accommodate you in this matter. You can also let the person in charge of meal appointments for missionaries in the branch, ward, or stake in which you are serving know of these requests so they can relay the information to those members who sign-up to feed you. Be thankful for whatever food you are served. Focus on the foods that are healthy and eat more of them, while avoiding or eating only a small portion of the foods that are not as healthy.

To avoid eating too much food at members' homes, eat slowly and always leave a little food on your plate. If your plate is empty and there is still plenty of time left during the appointment, they will think you want more food but are hesitant to ask, so they might offer you more food or take it upon themselves to dish you more!

It is a special occasion for members to have the missionaries in their homes for a meal so they will typically provide a dessert. Although the members may only eat one or two desserts all week with their meals, missionaries may eat dessert every night of the week at a different member's home. Eating dessert every night on your mission will compromise your healthy diet and may cause unhealthy weight gain. To avoid eating dessert, let members know you are in a hurry to get to your next appointment and must either skip dessert or take it with. Often-times you will also be offered to take extra food home. When this happens, work this food into your meal-plan for a later meal, give it to someone else who is in need of food, save it for your 10% cheat times (this will be discussed later), or if it totally compromises your nutritional program, dispose of it altogether.

Encourage members to invite a non-member friend, neighbor, or family member to the meal. Spend only 45 to

60 minutes at members' homes for meals. At the end of the meal, always show your gratitude by leaving a note or verbally expressing your thanks. Share a spiritual message with the family, commit them to do something to help with the missionary work in the area, and leave with a prayer. Above all else, be polite and sensitive to the feelings of the members when it comes to eating in their homes.

Emotional and non-hunger eating: Mission life, especially early on, is a roller coaster of emotions. In this situation, food can take on functions other than simply providing the body with nutrients and energy. Food can serve to distract or comfort, it may become a crutch or just something familiar to embrace. Using food to cope, celebrate, relax, or procrastinate are all examples of emotional or non-hunger eating. Everyone has eaten when they were not hungry, but the ability to manage these times is the key to avoiding unnecessary weight-gain.

Before you eat, decide whether you are really hungry. Are you eating because your body needs nourishment or for some other reason? Do not reward yourself with food. Most missionaries will want to celebrate after a baptism or after achieving another significant accomplishment or milestone on their mission. Celebrations traditionally revolve around food. If you are struggling with healthy eating, you might consider finding an alternative to celebrating with food. Try rewarding yourself in other ways. For example, do an activity you have wanted to do on the following preparation day.

Avoid eating when stressed. A lot of people turn to food during times of stress, which, for a missionary, is almost daily. Replace this food-eating response with a more positive behavior such as meditating, studying the gospel, reading scriptures, or praying.

Grocery shopping: Make sure you buy and stock your kitchen with healthy and nutritious foods. By doing so, you will always be prepared to eat healthy meals and you will be less tempted to eat unhealthy alternatives. If you do not buy unhealthy foods, you will not be able to eat them.

EAT EVERY 2-3 HOURS

When you eat is just as important as what you eat. Growing up most people heard the recommendation to eat three square meals a day and avoid eating anything in between meals for fear of ruining their appetite. Experts now agree these old beliefs are more detrimental to a person's health. You need to eat regularly to supply the body with a steady and regular flow of nutrients. By going too long between eating, you are more likely to lose muscle mass and develop body fat.

This way of eating slows the metabolism causing the body to break down muscle tissue for energy. It increases the amount of food you eat at each sitting, forcing the body into an unnatural state, storing most of what you eat as fat. Eating in this manner will also increase stress hormone production and decreases the body's ability to manage blood-sugar levels leading to chronic fatigue.

It is much healthier to consume several small, well-balanced meals every two to three hours. This should give you at least six feeding opportunities throughout the day. By no means should you eat a full, complete meal each time! Three of the feeding opportunities should be similar to a regular meal while the other three should be more like a healthy snack or "mini-meals."

DRINK WATER

The Apostle John wrote, "In the last day, that great

day of the feast, Jesus stood and cried, saying if any man thirst, let him come unto me, and drink. He that believeth on me, as the scripture hath said, out of his belly shall flow rivers of living water" (John 7:37-38).

Partaking of living water is necessary to sustain more than just spiritual life. It is also essential to physical survival. Humans can live for a few weeks without food, but only a few days without water. Water is the most abundant substance on earth and the most prevalent substance in the human body. It is the foundation of every physiological function performed in the body including digestion, circulation, and elimination. Proper hydration, improves the efficiency of the cardiovascular system, transports vital nutrients throughout the body, carries toxic wastes from the body, aids in injury prevention and recovery by protecting internal organs and tissues, lubricates joints making them last longer, and even regulates body temperature keeping all organs and tissues in optimal working condition. The body needs a constant supply of water because it is continuously lost through perspiration, evaporation, respiration, and waste. A lack of hydration causes sluggishness, dulled senses, stalled muscle growth and recovery, a general feeling of fatigue, a build-up of toxic wastes in the body, and a lack of overall performance.

Here are some guidelines to ensure you are getting a sufficient amount of water on a daily basis:

Most people should try to consume about sixty-four ounces of clean, pure, and fresh water every day. However, missionaries lead a more active and physical life, so perhaps you should drink up to ten, eight-ounce glasses of water a day. If you serve in a hot and/or humid climate you should drink even more water because warmer climates and physical activity increase your hydration needs.

One of the best ways to ensure you are drinking enough water is to drink two, eight-ounce glasses of water first thing in the morning upon arising, and then each hour after that drink anywhere from four to eight-ounces of water. If you follow this schedule you should have no problem with your water intake.

Purchase a backpack with a pouch or sleeve to hold a water hydration reservoir that you can carry with you providing a convenient and readily available source of water while performing your daily responsibilities as a missionary. These packs can also double as a regular backpack to carry scriptures, teaching materials, and meals while you are away from your apartment. If a water hydration backpack is not an option, then at the very least, you should have a high-quality water bottle that you can bring wherever you go. Whichever method you choose, be sure to fill it with fresh water each morning before you leave for the day. Add a lemon or lime wedge to your water to help kill bacteria and give the water a nice twist of flavor.

Finding clean water to drink can be an issue in some missions. If you are serving in one of these missions, make sure you drink only bottled water that has an unbroken seal. Drink water from reputable and reliable sources. Never use tap water for drinking, brushing your teeth, cleaning your fruits and vegetables, and avoid putting ice cubes in your drinks.

Jesus told the woman at the well that she would never thirst again if she drank the water He gave her (see John 4:10). The woman at the well learned a valuable lesson and she was so full of joy, she ran to share the message with others. As a missionary you are doing just that. You are offering living water to those who are thirsting spiritually. Make sure your physical thirst is regularly satisfied so you can continue to help those who thirst spiritually.

EAT NATURAL, WHOLE FOODS

God created a natural source of life-giving food for His children. These foods, in their original state provide all the nutrients the body needs to sustain a healthy life. Natural, whole-foods, the way God intended them to be, promote health and wellness. In general, the more natural and less-refined the foods you eat are, the healthier you will be. God's ways are perfect, pure, and balanced. These foods were approved as "very good" by God Himself (see Genesis 1:31) and can not be improved upon by man.

Unfortunately, food manufacturers have grossly altered many of these natural foods in an effort to make them more convenient, cheaper, last longer on store shelves, and look more attractive. They are usually prepackaged, found in a bag, a box, or a can and are often void of color, or infused with artificial coloring. Processed foods promote disease and sickness. The more processes a food goes through, the more damage it causes the body and the less nutrition the body receives. Sadly, these foods have been so robbed of their life-giving qualities that they are a perversion of what God intended them to be! Avoid these foods and feed your body instead with unprocessed, natural foods as much as possible.

EAT VEGETABLES AT EACH MEAL

Vegetables are high in nutrition and low in calories. They are packed full of vitamins and minerals which are essential to good health. Vitamins are responsible for growth, regulating the energy you get from food, and protecting against disease. Minerals are building blocks for bones, they help muscles contract and relax, initiate chemical reactions in the body, and help nerves transmit messages. Vegetables are also high in fiber which aids in keeping the digestive tract healthy. You should include at least one serving of vegetables with each meal.

Buy fresh vegetables in season whenever possible and try to buy locally grown produce, assuming you are in a mission where this is permitted. Some missions are in areas of the world where the fruit and vegetable farmers do not abide by healthy growing methods, harming the produce they grow, causing sickness or disease. Look to your mission president for guidance if you suspect you may be in one of these areas.

EAT PROTEIN AT EACH MEAL

Protein is the building block to every cell in the body. Skin, bones, organs, hair, and muscles are all made up of proteins. Protein is responsible for many of the physiological functions in the body like fighting off infections and regulating hormone levels. Eat a serving of complete protein with every meal. Foods that are high in protein are more filling than foods high in carbohydrates and fats; and it takes more energy for the body to digest protein which increases the metabolism. Protein also slows the absorption of carbohydrates into the bloodstream preventing unnatural spikes in blood-sugar and insulin levels avoiding excess storage of body fat.

EAT A VARIETY OF HEALTHY FATS

Many people believe that all fat is bad. This is simply not true. Fat is essential to a healthy diet. Although there is a stigma about the fat in food, the body needs a certain amount of the right types of fat to perform basic physiological functions. Healthy fats are necessary in the diet in order to help the body produce energy, protect vital organs from damage, absorb certain essential vitamins, insulate from the cold, repair and grow tissues, regulate blood pressure, assist in fat metabolism, keep cell membranes fluid and flexible, neutralize the negative effects of unhealthy fats, keep inflammation of the joints and body tissue to a minimum, and reduce bad cholesterol.

Twenty-five to thirty-five percent of your diet should come from an equal blend of healthy fats. There are essentially three kinds of naturally occurring fats that should be consumed: saturated, monounsaturated, and polyunsaturated. Saturated fats come from animal sources such as meat, dairy products, and eggs. Monounsaturated fats come from mixed nuts, olives, and olive oil. Polyunsaturated fats come from flaxseed oil, fish oils, and mixed nuts. Consuming a healthy balance of all three will dramatically improve your overall health.

Avoid hydrogenated fats and trans-fatty acids whenever possible. They are the most dangerous fats, clogging blood vessels and creating imbalances in the body. These are unsaturated oils that have been chemically altered to be solid, instead of liquid, at room temperature and are found in shortening, margarine, unnatural peanut butter, and most baked goods.

CHEAT 10% OF THE TIME

Some of these strategies might seem a little overbearing or make you feel too restricted in your eating. Do not worry! Each week you will have a chance to eat and drink some of your favorite foods and beverages as long as you are adhering to the other strategies 90% of the time.

This is as much a psychological strategy as it is physical. By cheating 10% of the time you will relieve any psychological feelings of deprivation that may build-up throughout the week. This strategy keeps you from getting bored with your diet and allows you to eat foods that do not comply with the other strategies for those special occasions. Permitting yourself this flexibility allows you to enjoy certain foods without feeling guilty because it is part of your overall nutritional strategy. Believe it or not, by following this strategy you will actually burn more fat and build more muscle.

The general premise behind this strategy is to eat anything you want or skip any meal you want up to 10% of the total meals eaten throughout the week. The easiest way to figure this out is to add up all the times you eat each day and multiply this by seven for the number of days in the week. Then take 10% of that number. For most missionaries, you should be eating about six times a day. Spread out over a full week this would be forty-two feeding opportunities. Ten percent of forty-two is approximately four. So as long as you keep your cheating to four times or less per week, you will not disrupt your overall health.

GET PLENTY OF FRESH AIR

"And the Lord God formed man of the dust of the ground, and breathed into his nostrils the breath of life; and man became a living soul" (Genesis 2:7). Without the breath of life humans would cease to live within a matter of minutes. The body is more dependent on oxygen than on any other nutrient, including water. You can live a few weeks without food, a few days without water, but only a few minutes without oxygen before irreversible damage occurs. Just as oxygen was necessary to bring Adam to life, it is also oxygen that is necessary to sustain life.

The quality of air you breathe affects the quality and length of life you live. Unfortunately, today's modern environment is so polluted that fresh air is limited. A lack of fresh air can leave you feeling nauseous, irritable, fatigued, tired, headachy, depressed, and stressed. Fortunately, there are a few things you can do in your own personal environment to help with the quality of air you breathe.

One of the simplest things you can do is to open windows in your apartment first thing in the morning to let fresh air in and to circulate the stale air out that accumulated overnight as you and your companion slept. Also bring a small plant into your apartment. It not only gives color and energy, but also helps freshen-up the air. Humans and plants have a symbiotic relationship. Humans exhale carbon dioxide and plants exhale oxygen as waste products. To sustain life, we use the oxygen from the plants and the plants use the carbon dioxide we produce.

Finally, when you are in an environment where it is not possible to always breathe clean, fresh air, you can still get sufficient amounts of oxygen by performing deep-breathing exercises regularly throughout the day. The proper way to perform deep-breathing exercises is to first, get into a position where you are standing or sitting-up with your back straight. Inhale through your nose slowly for a count of five. As you inhale, expand your rib cage and your abdomen and hold your breathe for a two-count. Finally exhale slowly through your mouth for a count of five or until you have exhaled as much air as possible. Hold this for a two-count and repeat the entire process three to five times. Perform this deep-breathing exercise as often as you get a chance throughout the day. By doing so you will be able to focus better, have more energy, and lessen the effect of stress on your body.

GET SUFFICIENT AMOUNTS OF SUNSHINE EACH DAY

All of God's creations are dependent, either directly or indirectly, on the nourishing rays of the sun. Light brings life. This is true in both the physical and spiritual realm. The sun supplies energy and warmth to the body just like the Son, or the Light of Christ, provides energy and soothing warmth to the soul.

You may have healthy food, sufficient rest, adequate exercise, and plenty of fresh air, but without sunlight you will not have complete health. Natural sunlight has a powerful healing affect on the body and spirit. W h e n you spend time in the sunlight, your body soaks in the life-giving elements the sun offers. Nerve endings close to the skin absorb the energy from the sun and send it through the body, relaxing, rejuvenating, and re-nourishing it.

As your health increases, you will have a natural desire for sunlight. The healthier you become, the more you will be attracted to things that are healthy and life-giving. Spend as much time, within reason, outside in the sunlight. During the spring and summer months try to get a minimum of ten-minutes of sunlight each day and in the fall and winter months get at least twenty-minutes of sunlight each day.

Too often missionaries try to do too much, too soon. Rarely is it possible to make a lot of changes in your life all at once and expect to succeed. In order to realistically implement these nutritional strategies you should make small, incremental changes to your diet by slowly adding one strategy at a time over a period of several months until each of them individually becomes a lasting habit. By making gradual changes, you will find it easier and more effective to sustain a healthy way of eating throughout your mission and your life.

SAMPLE MEAL-PLANS

Now, it is time to get practical! This section is designed to provide you with some sample meal-plans based on the strategies above.

MISSIONARY 1, APPROXIMATELY 140 lbs or Less (Goal: Muscle Gain/Maintenance)	
MEAL #1	Omelet 2 egg whites, 1 whole egg 1-2 servings vegetables 1/3 cup oatmeal 1 serving fruit
MEAL #2	Smoothie 1/2 cup mixed berries 1 tbsp almonds 1/2 cup nonfat, plain yogurt 1 cup orange juice, ice, or water
MEAL #3	Sandwich 3 oz extra-lean meat 2 slices whole-grain bread 2-3 servings vegetables 1 piece fruit
MEAL #4	1 piece fruit 1 oz light string cheese
MEAL #5	3 oz extra-lean meat 1/2 cup whole-wheat pasta or rice 2-3 servings vegetables
MEAL #6	1/3 cup nonfat, plain yogurt 1 tbsp mixed nuts

MISSIONARY 1, APPROXIMATELY 140 lbs or Less (Goal: Fat Loss)	
MEAL #1	Omelet 2 egg whites, 1 whole egg 2-3 servings vegetables
MEAL #2	1/2 cup low-fat cottage cheese 1 tbsp almonds (or protein shake)
MEAL #3	Salad 3 oz extra-lean meat 2-3 cups of spinach 2-3 servings vegetables 1 tbsp vinaigrette
MEAL #4	1 piece fruit 1 oz light string cheese
MEAL #5	3 oz extra-lean meat 1/2 cup whole-wheat pasta or rice 2-3 servings vegetables
MEAL #6	1/3 cup low-fat cottage cheese 1/2 tbsp almonds (or protein shake)

MISSIONARY 2, APPROXIMATELY 170 lbs (Goal: Muscle Gain/Maintenance)	
MEAL #1	Omelet 3 egg whites, 1 whole egg 2 servings vegetables 1/2 cup oatmeal 1 serving fruit
MEAL #2	Smoothie 3/4 cup mixed berries 2 tbsp almonds 3/4 cup non-fat, plain yogurt 1 cup orange juice, ice, or water
MEAL #3	Sandwich 4 oz extra-lean meat 2 slices whole-grain bread 3 servings vegetables 1 piece fruit
MEAL #4	1 piece fruit 2 oz light string cheese
MEAL #5	4 oz extra-lean meat 3/4 cup whole-wheat pasta or rice 3 servings vegetables
MEAL #6	1/2 cup non-fat, plain yogurt 1 tbsp mixed nuts

MISSIONARY 2, APPROXIMATELY 170 lbs (Goal: Fat Loss)	
MEAL #1	Omelet 3 egg whites, 1 whole egg 2 servings vegetables
MEAL #2	3/4 cup low-fat cottage cheese 2 tbsp almonds (or protein shake)
MEAL #3	Salad 4 oz extra-lean meat 2-3 cups spinach 3 servings vegetables 1 tbsp vinaigrette
MEAL #4	1 piece fruit 2 oz light string cheese
MEAL #5	4 oz extra-lean meat 3/4 cup whole-wheat pasta or rice 3 servings vegetables
MEAL #6	1/2 cup low-fat cottage cheese 3/4 tbsp almonds (or protein shake)

MISSIONARY 3, APPROXIMATELY 200 lbs or More (Goal: Muscle Gain/Maintenance)	
MEAL #1	Omelet 3 egg whites, 1 whole egg 2 servings vegetables 3/4 cup oatmeal 1 serving fruit
MEAL #2	Smoothie 1 cup mixed berries 2 tbsp almonds 1 cup non-fat, plain yogurt 1 cup orange juice, ice, or water
MEAL #3	Sandwich 5-6 oz extra-lean meat 2 slices whole-grain bread 3-4 servings vegetables 1 piece fruit
MEAL #4	1 piece fruit 2 oz light string cheese
MEAL #5	5-6 oz extra-lean meat 1 cup whole-wheat pasta or rice 3-4 servings vegetables
MEAL #6	3/4 cup non-fat, plain yogurt 1 tbsp mixed nuts

MISSIONARY 3, APPROXIMATELY 200 lbs or More (Goal: Fat Loss)	
MEAL #1	Omelet 3 egg whites, 1 whole egg 2 servings vegetables
MEAL #2	1 cup low-fat cottage cheese 2 tbsp almonds (or protein shake)
MEAL #3	Salad 5-6 oz extra-lean meat 2-3 cups spinach 3-4 servings vegetables 1 tbsp vinaigrette
MEAL #4	1 piece fruit 2 oz light string cheese
MEAL #5	5-6 oz extra-lean meat 1 cup whole-wheat pasta or rice 3-4 servings vegetables
MEAL #6	3/4 cup low-fat cottage cheese 1 tbsp almonds (or protein shake)

Healthy dietary habits can positively influence your success as a missionary. Begin early and learn as much as you can about proper nutrition before leaving on your mission. By so doing, you can more effectively implement these nutritional strategies and modify the sample meal-plans to accommodate your individual needs. For quick and easy recipes that apply the nutritional strategies found in this chapter, please refer to the companion cookbook to this book titled: *Missionary Fitness Cookbook*, available at www.missionaryfitness.com.

NOURISHING
YOUR SPIRIT

It is impossible to ignore the body's need for constant nutrients. The physical body has built-in mechanisms, such as hunger pangs and thirst, to let you know when it needs more nutrients. The constant need for nutrients to sustain the spirit is much less obvious, but equally important. As a result the spiritual nourishment tends to be neglected and sometimes even ignored. This can escalate to spiritual malnutrition and eventually leads to spiritual deficiencies. Nutrients required by the spirit on a regular basis include prayer, scripture and gospel study, service to others, and, perhaps one of the most powerful, fasting.

"Fasting, a voluntary abstinence from food, is a principle of the gospel of Jesus Christ for developing spiritual strength; it has always existed among true believers" (Bible Dictionary, 671). Many great miracles found in the scriptures came as a result of faithful prayer and fasting – from Jesus (see Matthew 4:2) to Moses (see Exodus 34:28), and from Elijah (see 1 Kings 19:8) to Alma and the sons of Mosiah (see Alma 17:3). When you fast on your mission, in some ways, you re-enact the fast performed by these mighty men and consequently, you will witness many miracles of your own, just as they did.

Here are several strategies you should employ when fasting in order to help you satisfy your spiritual appetite and experience many great miracles while on your mission.

DECIDE ON A PURPOSE FOR YOUR FAST

There are many reasons for which you can fast. You might fast to receive divine guidance, revelation, or answers to questions; to grow closer to God; to weaken the power Satan has in your life; to cope with difficulties; to gain freedom from bondage (addictions); to develop spiritual strength; to increase control over the physical body; to be relieved of heavy burdens; to break through a depression or rut in life; to seek God's face; to increase faith and self-confidence; to be freed from temptations; to have more power to resist temptations; to have a clear and focused mind; to bring peace and comfort; or to have humility.

Fasting can also help you establish self-control; eliminate bad eating habits; slow the aging process; increase physical and spiritual strength; breakdown stored body fat; eliminate body odor and bad breath; clear the skin and brighten the eyes; eliminate chronic fatigue; clear up foggy or fuzzy thinking; elevate self-esteem; relieve stress, anxiety, and tension; and allow for better sleep.

All of these reasons to fast can, essentially, be narrowed down into three main categories. The physical purposes, the spiritual purposes, and the purpose to provide help for those in need.

Physical Purpose of Fasting

The two main physical purposes that fasting serves for the body are to give the internal organs a rest and to cleanse the body of wastes and toxic build-up. The body is designed to enjoy regular periods of rest from physical labor each night. The internal organs deserve, and even require, the same rest each night in order to function optimally. Every morning when you awake and eat the first meal of the day, you are essentially breaking a fast by eating "break-fast." In similar fashion, we are commanded to work six days a week and rest on the seventh. The internal organs also need an equal ratio of work and rest to properly perform their functions. The law of rest applies universally to all aspects of the physical body, including the internal organs. The following scripture illustrates this point, "this is a day appointed to pay thy devotions to the most high; And on this day thou shalt do none other thing, only let thy food be prepared with singleness of heart that thy fasting may be perfect" (D&C 59:10, 13). A meal prepared with "singleness of heart" not only prevents working unnecessarily on the Sabbath, but also provides for a simple meal, which is easier for the internal organs to digest and assimilate.

Fasting allows the body to direct its energy toward other, often neglected functions, rather than digesting and assimilating food. The body can focus on cleansing, purifying, and in some cases, healing tissue and organ cells. This brief period of rest helps the body catch up on maintenance and repair work, replenish enzymes, restore proper balance, and eliminate accumulated waste, poisons, and toxic build-up.

As you give the internal organs the rest they need, the cleaner and healthier they will become. The cleaner and healthier they become, the cleaner and healthier your body will become. The cleaner and healthier your body becomes, the cleaner and healthier your spirit becomes.

Spiritual Purpose of Fasting

Despite the powerful physical purposes for fasting, the spiritual purposes are far more significant. The law of fasting is a gift from God to assist His children in growing closer to Him and gaining a greater understanding of His ways. Fasting breaks the bondage of physical appetites and desires. It promotes spiritual development by creating an atmosphere where the flesh is coerced into submission by the spirit. Once this occurs, the Holy Ghost can work more powerfully in your life allowing a whole new opportunity for growth.

Bruce R. McConkie said, "Fasting, with prayer as its companion, is designed to increase spirituality; to foster a spirit of devotion and love of God; to increase faith in the hearts of men, thus assuring divine favor; to encourage humility and contrition of soul; to aid in the acquirement of righteousness; to teach man his nothingness and dependence on God; and to hasten those who properly comply with the law of fasting along the path of salvation" (McConkie, *Mormon Doctrine*, 276).

Providing Help for Those in Need

An added benefit of fasting, whether fasting for a physical purpose or a spiritual purpose, allows you to provide help to those in need through fast offerings. President Spencer W. Kimball taught, "This principle of promise, when lived in the spirit thereof, greatly blesses both the giver and receiver. Upon practicing the law of the fast, one finds a personal well-spring of power to overcome self-indulgence and selfishness" (Kimball, 145). The money you save from not eating the food you normally would have, should be given as fast offerings which are used to help those in need.

As a missionary, you are exempt from paying tithing because you are not earning any kind of income. However, you are still expected to pay a generous fast offering, because you will still go without food and drink for a period of time saving you the money you otherwise would have spent. In fact, the Missionary Handbook states, "You can gain the full blessings of the law of the fast by paying fast offerings on fast Sunday to the bishop or branch president where you are serving" (*Missionary Handbook*, 32). Know that fasting with a purpose, whatever that purpose may be, can result in greater spiritual and physical rewards.

PLAN AND PREPARE FOR YOUR FAST

Just as you must plan and prepare for your physical food intake, you must also plan and prepare for your fast.

In the day or two leading up to your fast, be very strict with your diet. Focus on eating fresh fruits and vegetables; try to avoid meat and other animal products, and stay away from pre-packaged, processed, and fast-food. By doing this, the fast will be easier for you to accomplish and much easier on your body. Also be sure to get plenty of rest the night before the fast is to begin, or in some cases, the night the fast actually begins.

Prior to beginning the fast, decide on an appropriate amount for fast offerings and prepare to have that amount ready to give to the bishop or branch president in the area you are serving. This way you do not need to spend time making this monetary decision on the day of the fast, taking away from the fast itself.

Schedule the day of your fast so you will have sufficient time to pray, ponder, and study concerning the purpose of your fast. If possible, it is best to schedule the day of your fast on a day where there will be minimal output of physical energy. Typically, this is why fasting is done on the Sabbath day – the day of rest. However, you are not limited to fasting only on the Sabbath. Just make sure if you fast on any other day, you limit your physical activity as much as possible; otherwise it may be a challenge to get through the day. If necessary and appropriate, you might need to let your companion or others know of your intent to fast and the duration of the fast. By letting them know, they will be mindful of your situation and the needs that go along with it.

During your fast and the few days following, you may experience symptoms associated with cleansing and the elimination of toxins and wastes from your body. Some of the symptoms you may experience are: headaches, nausea, weakness, dizziness, lightheadedness, restlessness, disturbed sleep, cramping, chills, and/or achy joints and muscles. These symptoms should not be cause for alarm. However, if any of these symptoms persist for a prolonged period of time, you should seek assistance from a medical professional.

Fasting is a process and Heavenly Father does not expect you to be an expert at it the first time, or even after the first several times you attempt it. There will be times when you are not able to complete a fast for the previously decided upon duration. If this occurs, do not let it get you down – no one is keeping score – it is not a contest. Next time, simply plan and prepare the best you can and strive to accomplish the duration you decide upon, continually seeking strength through prayer in order to accomplish it.

DETERMINE THE TYPE AND LENGTH OF YOUR FAST

For the purpose of this discussion, there are two main types of fasting: a complete or absolute fast and a partial fast. A complete or absolute fast is what most people commonly think of as a fast. It is where you do not eat or drink anything for a pre-determined period of time. This is the most intense form of fasting. This type of fasting is best exemplified in the scriptures by Jesus, Moses, and Elijah. Each of them went without food or drink for forty-days. The fasting demonstrated by these great men proved their desire for spiritual issues super-ceded their desire for physical appetites. Although the fast performed by them was for forty full days, you do not need to, nor should you perform a fast for such a long duration in order to receive the blessings that come from fasting.

The first thing you should do after deciding on a purpose for your fast should be to decide how long the fast will last. This is important to know at the beginning because it will help prepare you mentally and physically for what will come and you will be much better prepared to accomplish your fast if you have an idea of when it will end. Be realistic in deciding how long the fast should be. Typically, the longer the fast, the more planning and preparation should go into it. Keep in mind that as a missionary there are guidelines and restrictions on your fasting. The Missionary Handbook instructs that, "Occasionally you may fast for a special reason, but the fast should not extend beyond one day. Generally, the monthly fast is sufficient" (*Missionary Handbook*, 32).

A fast is typically thought to last for a period of twenty-four hours. Although this is a sufficient amount of time to fast, a fast does not always need to be this long to be beneficial. Evidence for this is given by Joseph F. Smith: "I say to my brethren, when they are fasting and praying for the sick and for those who need faith and prayer, do not go beyond what is wise and prudent in fasting and prayer. The Lord can hear a simple prayer offered in faith, in half a dozen words, and he will recognize fasting that may not continue more than twenty-four hours just as readily and as effectively as he will answer a prayer of a thousand words and fasting for a month" (Smith, *Conference Report*, 133-134).

Perhaps the best method for participating in a twenty-four hour fast is to no longer eat after dinner the night you begin your fast; usually this is a Saturday night. Do not eat or drink anything the following day as well, typically a Sunday. Toward the conclusion of the fast, prior to dinner on the day of the fast, end your fast with a prayer and break it with a simple meal. You should already have this meal made so you can just warm it up and finalize the preparation with a "singleness of heart." Otherwise you risk spending too much time and energy on the meal, detracting from the real purpose of the day.

The second type of fast is a partial fast. This type of fast allows the person fasting to consume only certain, pre-determined foods or beverages in a limited amount. It may mean abstaining from just one meal a day, abstaining from a certain type of food, abstaining from all solid foods and drinking only liquids for a period of time, or only preparing meals with a "singleness of heart" (see D&C 59:13). In this sense "every Sabbath should be a fast day" (Smith & Sjodahl, 352).

Unfortunately, in the LDS social tradition, "Sunday dinner" is an event where all of the family gathers together to consume the largest meal of the week. Preparing for and consuming such a feast is labor-intensive and detracts from the real purpose of the Sabbath. This point is clearly illustrated in a revelation given to the prophet Joseph Smith: "And on this day thou shalt do none other thing, only let thy food be prepared with singleness of heart that thy fasting may be perfect, or, in other words, that thy joy may be full" (D&C 59:13).

If a special meal is to be served on the Sabbath, most of the preparation, if not all, should be done prior to the

Sabbath day. Even if it is prepared prior to the Sabbath, the meal which is to be consumed should be relatively simple so that the digestive organs do not need to work anymore than necessary to properly digest the food. This also detracts from the real purpose of the Sabbath day by deflecting a lot of energy towards the digestive process rather than on strengthening the spirit and growing closer to God.

BEGIN YOUR FAST WITH A PRAYER

Fasting and prayer go hand-in-hand. Rarely is fasting mentioned in the scriptures without mention of prayer. Essentially this is because going without food or drink for a period of time without a purpose or the accompaniment of prayer is not fasting at all – it is simply going hungry. Avoiding food or drink alone will unnecessarily starve your body and weaken you physically, doing you no good spiritually.

Soon after your last meal, prior to beginning your fast, you should find a quiet and private place to kneel down and pray. This prayer will officially mark the beginning of your fast. Include thanks and gratitude for your blessings and express your desires and purpose for the fast. You may also need to ask for physical strength and stamina to help you get through the fast. Then quietly meditate and listen for any promptings you may receive from the spirit. Finally, you should appropriately end your prayer in the name of Jesus Christ because it is by and through Him that all things are possible, including fasting.

ACTIVITIES TO DO DURING YOUR FAST

During your fast you should always maintain the spirit while directing your thoughts and actions toward the purpose of your fast. Always be open and willing to let God direct your fast. Following are some important activities you can do during your fast to maintain the Spirit and focus more fully on the purpose of your fast.

Dedicate the extra time you save from preparing and eating meals to participating in inspiring and uplifting activities such as praying, pondering, serving others, taking a walk outdoors in the fresh air and sunlight, writing in your journal, jotting down your thoughts and feelings, and reading the scriptures. One particular scripture you can read and study during your fast is Isaiah chapter 58. This chapter is dedicated to explaining the proper way to fast and is great at explaining the numerous blessings that come as a result of fasting.

If you are fasting on a Sunday, be sure to attend all of your church meetings. You might also find it helpful to attend firesides, devotionals, or other uplifting and inspiring meetings as long as they are directly related to your missionary work. When you participate in these activities, your body and spirit will receive nourishment in other ways and your mind will be distracted from the physical pains that are sometimes associated with fasting.

As your fast progresses you may begin to experience thirst and hunger pangs. You may even begin to feel weak and tired. If this occurs follow the counsel of Jesus, "Moreover when ye fast, be not, as the hypocrites, of a sad countenance: for they disfigure their faces, that they may appear unto men to fast. Verily I say unto you, they have their reward. But thou, when thou fastest, anoint thine head, and wash thy face; That thou appear not unto men to fast, but unto thy father which is in secret: and thy father, which seeth in secret, shall reward thee openly" (Matthew 6:16-18).

END YOUR FAST WITH A PRAYER AND BREAK IT WITH A SIMPLE MEAL

By the end of your fast you may feel physically tired, but you should feel spiritually refreshed. As you prepare to end your fast, spend some time alone in a quiet room and listen to the spirit. It is important to plan for this time because often the answer or solution to the purpose of your fast will come at the very end of your fast. However, be prepared because sometimes it does not come until long after the fast is over.

After you have spent some time alone pondering, and once you feel ready, you should end your fast in the same manner as you began – with prayer. Be sure to express gratitude and thanks for the opportunity to fast, growing closer to Heavenly Father and feeling of His love. Express gratitude for His help with the purpose for which you fasted and express your desire for continued help and support in this endeavor.

Although you have "ended" the fast with a prayer, the process of fasting is not completely over. Ending your fast is a two-step process. First, you must end your fast with a prayer and second, you must break your fast with a meal. How you break the fast is physically just as important as the fast itself.

The most common mistake people make when breaking a fast is to eat too much, too quickly. As you fast, your stomach decreases in size limiting the amount of food you can eat. Also the body reacts very strongly to the food you ingest following a fast. If the food is good, high-quality food, the body reacts in a positive manner. If the food is of poor quality, then the body will react in a negative manner. Certain foods tend to be harder on the body after a fast. As a result, you should stay away from processed foods, junk food, fast-food, and even animal-based food products when breaking your fast. The best option is to break the fast with raw or lightly steamed vegetables and fruits. Above all else, the most important thing to remember when eating the first meal after fasting is to take your time and stay in control by overcoming the temptation to eat too much.

Relatively soon after ending your fast with a prayer and breaking it with a simple meal, it is a good idea to shower or bathe. During a fast your body releases toxins and wastes through the pores in the skin. Bathing will help wash them off of your skin so they do not cause problems with bacterial growth, which can cause body odor, irritation of the skin, acne, and infections.

REFLECT ON YOUR FAST OFTEN

During the period of time after your fast ends and before you begin to think about your next fast, you should have plenty of time to reflect on the impressions and events that occurred during the fast. Ponder on the purpose of your fast and how it was accomplished. Think about what went well and what you could have improved. Read the journal entry or notes you jotted down from your last fast to remember the thoughts and feelings you experienced. Consider how you have grown spiritually. Reflect on all of this often as a source of spiritual strength.

Fasting is not a time of deprivation, but rather a time of spiritual growth – a way to overcome the body's natural appetites while helping others in the process. It is a privilege and is something you should look forward to. Most importantly, it is a powerful way to experience complete spiritual and physical health.

FIT FOR SERVICE, PART I:
Understanding The Basics

Proper nutrition can not prepare your body and spirit alone. However, proper nutrition combined with regular physical exercise will dramatically improve your ability to prepare your body and spirit in as short amount of time as possible. God created man to be physically active. The human body functions properly and optimally when it is exposed to physical movement on a regular basis. From the beginning of time when Adam and Eve were in the Garden of Eden, they were required to put forth some physical effort to eat and maintain their surroundings. In fact one of the earliest instructions God gave man was to be physically active as illustrated in the following scriptures:

"And the Lord God took the man, and put him into the Garden of Eden to dress it and keep it" (Genesis 2:15). And after the Fall "thorns and thistles" (see Genesis 3:18) afflicted the vegetation. This required an increase of physical effort to bring forth fruits and vegetables amid the oppressive weeds that were meant to torment man. "Therefore the Lord God sent him forth from the Garden of Eden, to till the ground from whence he was taken" (Genesis 3:23).

Man has been required to exert a great deal of physical effort just to sustain life by laboring for his food since the time Adam and Eve were expelled from the Garden of Eden until relatively recently. Over the last 100 years this has changed dramatically due to modern advancement in technology.

The modern world is now one of convenience and ease. However, this convenience and ease comes at a price. The daily physical activity of humans has significantly been reduced to such an extent that people no longer get the physical exercise their bodies need for optimal health.

There is nothing wrong with a modern world filled with labor-saving technologies as long as the work lost is replaced with sufficient physical activity from somewhere else. This can be accomplished through a daily exercise program.

In recent years Church leaders have recognized the importance of exercise on the health and morale of full-time missionaries. As a result the leaders have included 30-minutes of exercise into the daily missionary schedule.

If the counsel and instruction from Church leaders is not enough motivation for you to commit to exercise while on your mission, then here are some benefits from exercise that may help you understand its importance and convince you to include it in your daily life:

Daily exercise keeps your weight under control by increasing your muscle mass. The muscles of the body are like a furnace that burn fat for fuel. By exercising you can increase your muscle mass, which in turn, increases your metabolism and burns more fat during the day just to keep the increased muscles fueled.

Exercise increases muscle strength, giving you greater capacity to perform daily activities. Stronger muscles also provide better support for bones in the body, helping the body maintain proper positioning. Correct posture helps the body move more efficiently enabling it to perform daily activities with less stress and more ease. Exercise helps keep bones healthy and strong while slowing age-related bone loss.

Exercise keeps the body flexible; not only the muscles and connective tissue, but also the cells of the body. Body cells require daily stimulation to maintain pliability and elasticity. If they do not get this daily stimulation they will become weak, frail, and inefficient. Eventually, they will malfunction and slowly die causing a build-up of toxic waste in the body, which relates to the next benefit of exercise.

The lymphatic, or lymph, system rids the body of toxins and wastes and helps maintain the strength of the immune system. The lymph system does not have a pump to circulate lymph fluids through the body like the circulatory system has the heart to pump the blood. Instead, the lymph system relies solely on the body's movement, through muscle contractions to circulate the fluid. When the body does not move regularly, the lymph system loses its ability to move the waste and toxins out of the cells. When the lymphatic system backs up or becomes stagnant, due to a lack of exercise, the waste and toxins accumulate causing the immune system to weaken resulting in sickness and disease.

Exercise increases perspiration which is another method the body uses to rid itself of waste and toxins. Exercise helps the mind focus better by improving the circulation allowing more oxygenated blood to get to the brain. Exercise counters the conditions that lead to chronic diseases later in life by improving circulation, reducing the risk of heart disease, improving blood cholesterol, lowering high blood pressure, and preventing bone loss.

Daily exercise can produce more benefits than just physical fitness and health. It also promotes psychological well-being. It can promote feelings of accomplishment, self-confidence, and self-mastery, as well as improving your mood. It reduces stress and anxiety by releasing hormones naturally released during exercise. These hormones are classified as endorphins and they decrease pain, increase relaxation, release tension, counter anxiety and depression, improve quality of sleep, increase enthusiasm and optimism, and balance out the hormones brought on by stress.

Ultimately, consistent, daily exercise will help you strengthen and tone your muscles, burn fat, cleanse your body of toxic wastes, and slow the aging process, making you more energetic, healthy, youthful, confident, and properly balanced.

Before you can make and keep the commitment to exercise daily, you must first have a basic understanding of the elements that make up a well-designed exercise program in order to effectively transform your body and spirit.

ELEMENTS OF AN EXERCISE PROGRAM

A well-designed, general exercise program should consist of a combination of the following four elements: Dynamic Stretching, Energy System Training, Resistance Training, and Static Stretching.

Dynamic Stretching – Warming-Up to a Great Workout

The beginning of every exercise session needs to start with an effective warm-up in order to have a great workout. Warming-up prior to a workout has many benefits. A proper warm-up can increase your coordination, your work capacity, your body temperature, the blood flow to your heart and muscles, and the efficiency of your neuromuscular system. A proper warm-up also reduces the possibility of injury by making your muscles more pliable and improving the range of motion and lubrication in and around your joints. In addition, a proper warm-up can also reduce muscle soreness and joint stiffness.

In the past, the belief was that a warm-up prior to a workout should consist of a series of static stretches. Since then, numerous studies have concluded that this type of warm-up is inefficient. Not only can it increase your risk of injury, but it also sedates the nervous system and decreases your ability to get an effective workout. Static stretches designed to enhance flexibility should only be performed following your workout. This way flexibility can be enhanced without compromising the effectiveness of your workout.

The best warm-up prior to a workout should consist of a series of dynamic stretches. The term "dynamic" refers to the relatively slow, deliberate increase in the range of motion of your joints. A dynamic warm-up acts, essentially, as a transition from a lower-level of activity to a higher-level of activity. It should be long and intense enough to achieve freedom of movement in all working joints and tissues and should even cause mild perspiration, but not to the point of fatigue. Most people should be able to achieve an effective warm-up within 3 to 5 minutes.

Energy System Training – Serve with All Your Heart

Energy system training refers to your aerobic and anaerobic conditioning. The term aerobic means "with oxygen" and the term anaerobic means "without oxygen." Aerobic conditioning focuses on the health of the cardiovascular and respiratory systems and is characterized by any activity that involves continuous, rhythmic movement of large muscle groups at an increased heart rate of approximately 70% of the maximum heart rate for a minimum of 20 minutes. This type of exercise strengthens the heart, lungs, and blood vessels. It increases blood circulation, improves digestion and elimination, stimulates the lymphatic system, increases the production of neurotransmitters, and helps condition the body to circulate more oxygen to the brain and other organs and tissues more efficiently.

Anaerobic conditioning focuses on performing short-duration activities that are at relatively high intensity levels, requiring immediate energy. This type of training is important because of its application to performing regular, everyday activities such as walking up a couple flights of stairs, carrying the groceries in from the trunk of a car, or taking a heavy garbage can out to the curb.

Although, both aerobic and anaerobic exercises are important to developing good health, one form of anaerobic exercise can be more effective and efficient because it combines all of the health benefits of both forms of conditioning. It is known as high-intensity interval training and involves short bursts of moderate to high-intense activity followed by periods of longer-duration, less-intense activity. By using this training strategy more work can be performed in less time, with less overall fatigue. Another bonus to utilizing this type of training is that it will burn excess body-fat for a longer stretch of time than any other method while still preventing the breakdown of muscle tissue. It is for these reasons that the Missionary Fitness exercise program favors this type of energy system training.

Energy system training is so versatile because it can be performed with little or no exercise equipment and it can be performed indoors or outdoors. The best energy system exercises for missionaries are walking, running, cycling, stair climbing, and rope jumping because they require little, if any equipment.

For general physical fitness your energy system

training should be performed at least three times per week. If your goal is to burn excess body fat, you might consider increasing your energy system training to four or five sessions per week. For best results each energy system training workout should last from 20-25 minutes, not including the warm-up or cool-down.

Resistance Training – Serve with All Your Strength

Resistance training refers to exercises performed using some form of resistance to stimulate your muscles. Resistance training serves to increase muscle size, strength, power, or a combination of all three. Resistance training can also be used to increase flexibility, improve muscle imbalances that lead to bad posture, and improve your body's ability to cope with stress.

There are several forms of resistance that can be used when performing resistance exercises. The simplest, least-expensive, and most convenient form of resistance is your own bodyweight. It requires no equipment, no external resistance, and you can move from one exercise to the next relatively quickly and easily saving precious time and energy. This allows you to get more done in less time.

Regardless of your health and body transformation goals, you should be able to accomplish them by using primarily bodyweight exercises. If you are not convinced that your bodyweight will provide sufficient enough resistance for you to get a good workout, just take a look at any elite-level male gymnast. The majority of these gymnasts use only bodyweight exercises in their training and they have no problem developing great strength and powerful physiques.

The reason you can get such a great workout from your bodyweight alone is because it is possible to adjust the resistance your bodyweight provides by redistributing your weight between your limbs, manipulating the range of motion, performing the exercises in an unstable environment, varying the leverage, and minimizing bounce and momentum.

This is not to say that external resistance is not important, of course it is, but unless you can stabilize, control, and move your own bodyweight efficiently with excellent form for every exercise, then you have no reason to add external resistance. For this, and the fact that missionaries have very little, if any, exercise equipment, all of the resistance exercises illustrated in the next chapter can be performed using bodyweight only.

Once you can perform bodyweight exercises with proper form then you will be ready to implement external resistance into your workout. Exercise bands and tubing are a great form of external resistance for missionaries because they are lightweight, portable, and easy to pack, yet they provide a relatively high level of resistance. Like your own bodyweight, they are very effective at building muscle strength, endurance, power, and size if used correctly.

In addition to these basic forms of resistance, you may find that everyday objects can be a great source to use for resistance. Some examples are filling cans or jugs with water or sand, or filling a backpack with heavy books or rocks. You may even get lucky and find some old weights in your missionary apartment left there by previous missionaries. Just remember, if you accumulate such forms of resistance you must leave them behind when you transfer to a new area where you may have to start all over again finding or creating new forms of resistance.

For general physical fitness your resistance training should be performed at least three times per week. If your goal is to increase muscle mass then you might consider increasing your resistance training to four or five sessions per week. For best results each resistance training workout should last about 20-25 minutes not including the dynamic stretching warm-up and static stretching cool-down.

Static Stretching – Cooling-Down from a Great Workout

Static stretching is one of the best ways to cool down from a workout and should only be performed at the end of a workout. Static stretches are characterized by movements that are held in a stationary position for a relatively short amount of time (10-30 seconds). This type of stretching is typically the kind of stretching most people are familiar with. Static stretching improves quality of movement, promotes a balanced range-of-motion, increases flexibility, and decreases recovery time. It can also decrease susceptibility to injury and the formation of muscular adhesions.

VARIABLES OF AN EXERCISE PROGRAM

Regardless of your physical transformation goals, a well-designed exercise program should integrate several variables that must be carefully orchestrated to produce the results you are working toward. Following is a list and description of the variables used in the Missionary Fitness exercise program.

Frequency

Exercise frequency is defined as the number of exercise sessions performed each week. Heavenly Father is very clear with the number of days He expects us to participate in physical activities each week. "Six days shalt thou labour, and do all thy work: But the seventh day is the Sabbath of the Lord thy God" (Exodus 20:9-10).

So, an ideal exercise program design is one where you perform physical activity six days a week and rest on the seventh day. Six days of physical exercise is sufficient to achieve any physical transformation goals you may have. Performing physical exercise seven days in a row without a day of rest will eventually lead to injuries and a lack of progress due to overtraining.

The best approach to exercising six days a week, while targeting each element of an exercise program and without overtraining, is to perform energy system training three days a week and resistance training three days a week on alternating days with dynamic and static stretching integrated into each.

This approach to training will sufficiently train each of the major muscle movements and energy systems in the proper ratio, giving each adequate time to recover before being trained again.

The following is an example of what this workout schedule might look like:

	WEEK 1	WEEK 2
MONDAY	Total-body resistance workout A	Total-body resistance workout B
TUESDAY	Energy system workout	Energy system workout
WEDNESDAY	Total-body resistance workout B	Total-body resistance workout A
THURSDAY	Energy system workout	Energy system workout
FRIDAY	Total-body resistance workout A	Total-body resistance workout B
SATURDAY	Energy system workout	Energy system workout
SUNDAY	Rest	Rest

Here is another example of what your workout schedule might look like if you decide to train the major muscle movements of the upper-body and the major muscle movements of the lower-body on alternating days:

	WEEK 1	WEEK 2
MONDAY	Upper-body resistance workout	Lower-body resistance workout
TUESDAY	Energy system workout	Energy system workout
WEDNESDAY	Lower-body resistance workout	Upper-body resistance workout
THURSDAY	Energy system workout	Energy system workout
FRIDAY	Upper-body resistance workout	Lower-body resistance workout
SATURDAY	Energy system workout	Energy system workout
SUNDAY	Rest	Rest

Each week, thereafter, you should continue to follow this alternating pattern. It really does not matter if you start the week with a resistance workout or an energy system workout as long as you strive to maintain this pattern each week throughout the duration of your mission for the sake of consistency.

The sample program outlined in the next chapter utilizes the total-body workout split. Therefore, if you choose to follow an upper-body and lower-body workout split you will need to adjust the exercises accordingly.

Duration

Unfortunately, as a missionary, you have only a limited amount of time dedicated to exercise. Fortunately, thirty-minutes is just enough time to maintain, and even improve your health, fitness, and body composition, provided, of course, you use the right exercise program. In order to make the most of those thirty-minutes you need to be focused and on-task every single minute. Otherwise, you will needlessly waste your time and fail to accomplish the results you are seeking.

If, for some reason, you feel you need to exercise a little more, you might consider waking up a little earlier to allow more time without imposing on the rest of your schedule. Remember, however, if you do plan to wake up earlier you need to be able to function optimally on less sleep, or else you will need to go to bed a little earlier to receive the necessary amount of sleep. Before trying this you will need to get permission from your mission president. Additionally, you should never extend your exercise time by infringing on other activities planned in your daily schedule. If you do this, you will compromise your effectiveness as a missionary and the missionary work as a whole causing you to miss out on spiritual and physical blessings.

Exercise Selection

You must be selective in the exercises you choose to perform since your time and resources are limited. Each exercise needs to easily integrate into the unique missionary lifestyle by utilizing a small amount of space, use little or no equipment, maximize the effect of each exercise, and provide the most benefit to your health and fitness.

Generally, the more muscles involved when performing an exercise the more effective and beneficial the exercise. Rather than performing exercises that train individual muscle groups, wasting a lot of time and receiving little benefit, you should include compound, multi-joint movement patterns that incorporate several muscle groups in your resistance training program. These exercises provide the maximum benefit for the minimal amount of time available to exercise.

Also, these exercises are more functional and applicable to "real life." In everyday life you rarely use just one muscle to perform a particular function. When performing a single, daily activity you use several muscle groups working together as a functional unit in a movement pattern. For favorable results your exercise program needs to reflect this concept.

The chart on the following page is a list of the major movement patterns included in the Missionary Fitness exercise program with examples of corresponding exercises.

Exercise Order

The order in which you perform your exercises can have a significant impact on how well your body responds to the exercise program.

"For it must needs be, that there is an opposition in all things" (2 Nephi 2:11). The Law of Opposition applies to physical exercise just as it does to every other aspect of life. A majority of your daily activities utilize the same movement patterns and muscle groups on a repetitive basis, leaving the opposing movements and muscles under-used leading to muscle imbalances in the body. To reverse these imbalances and prevent unnecessary injuries and postural problems your resistance training program should incorporate exercises that work opposing movement patterns and muscle groups.

When performing exercises that work the movement

MOVEMENT PATTERNS	EXERCISES
Quad-dominant movements	Squat and lunge variations
Hip-dominant movements	Deadlift variations, glute/ham raise, and lying hip extension
Horizontal pushing movements	Pushup and chest press variations
Horizontal pulling movements	Lying back row and other rowing variations
Vertical pushing movements	Shoulder press variations, pike pushup, handstand pushup
Vertical pulling movements	Pull-up variations
Arm pushing movements	Triceps extension variations, chair dips
Arm pulling movements	Biceps curl variations
CORE MOVEMENTS	
Stabilization	Plank variations
Rotational	Abdominal twist variations
Trunk/Hip flexion	Abdominal sit-up, crunch, and reverse crunch variations
Trunk/Hip extension	Back extension and reverse back extension variations

patterns and muscle groups in opposition you allow the antagonistic muscles (non-working muscles) to be inhibited. They are completely relaxed and at rest. This is called reciprocal inhibition. For example, a pulling movement such as an arm curl, which uses the biceps, is considered an agonist to the triceps, which are the antagonists and are completely relaxed. This inhibition is like giving the antagonist muscles a quick nap allowing you to do twice as many exercises in the same amount of time while still receiving adequate recovery for all the muscles involved in each movement.

The resistance training portion of the Missionary Fitness exercise program given in the next chapter will pair the opposing movement patterns together so they are performed one right after the other. By doing exercises in this manner you would do one set of an exercise then quickly move to the opposing exercise performing one set before moving on to a second set of the first exercise. These opposing exercises are paired together using the indications of A1, A2; B1, B2; C1, C2; and so on.

Another important key with exercise order is to always start your resistance training workouts by working the movement patterns with the largest muscle groups first followed by each movement pattern that utilizes subsequently smaller muscle groups. For example you would exercise your larger back and chest muscles before exercising your smaller arm muscles.

Sets and Reps

Sets and reps are the "nuts and bolts" of a resistance training program. Reps refer to the number of repetitions performed with each exercise without resting, while sets are groups of these repetitions. So, for 3 sets of 10 reps, or more commonly written 3 x 10, you would perform 10 repetitions a total of 3 times with rest periods in between each set for a total of 30 reps. Sets and reps will vary depending on your individual goals.

Below is a general breakdown of how many sets and reps you should perform to help you achieve your individual goals.

GOAL	INCREASE STRENGTH	INCREASE MUSCLE SIZE	DECREASE BODY FAT & GENERAL PHYSICAL FITNESS
SETS	5 +	3	2-3
REPS	3-5	6-12	12 +

Intensity

Intensity is one of the most powerful variables when it comes to your exercise program because it can be changed relatively easily. Intensity usually refers to the amount of resistance or weight used for an exercise. But, in the case of energy system training, intensity can be described as a level of exertion.

For resistance training exercises, as you progress through your workouts and as the resistance begins to get easier, you have a couple of options to increase the resistance. First, you can increase the weight used for the exercise, although this option might not always be possible because of your situation as a missionary. Second, if the first alternative is not an option, you can follow these suggestions for making any resistance you may have feel heavier, even if it is just your bodyweight.

• Increase the amount of time performing the eccentric (lowering) phase of the exercise

- Increase the length of pause between the eccentric (lowering) and concentric (raising) phases of the exercise

- Use a pre-fatigued sequence where you fatigue the muscle doing other exercises first

- Use isometric (holding a contracted muscle) pauses during the toughest position of the exercise for 4 or 5 seconds

- Use one-and-a-half reps: Perform the eccentric phase, then perform one-quarter of the concentric phase, pause, return to the start of the concentric phase, pause, then complete the entire concentric phase

- Use one-and-a-quarter reps: Perform the entire rep, and then perform an additional quarter rep in the toughest part of the exercise

- Use an extremely wide grip/stance or an extremely narrow grip/stance while performing the exercise

- Perform a limited-range movement only, usually at the toughest point of the exercise

- Train unilaterally, exercising only one limb at a time

- Perform oscillatory isometrics: Perform 4-5 short-range, mini-reps at the end-range of the exercise

- Ladder reps: Break the exercise up into thirds – the bottom third, the bottom 2/3rds, and the entire exercise and perform the number of reps you decide to do in the bottom third of the exercise, then perform that same number of reps in the bottom 2/3rds of the exercise, and finally, perform that same number of reps for the full-range of the exercise

You can perform any one, or combination, of these methods to make the resistance feel heavier.

For energy system training you should gauge the intensity of each workout on a scale of exertion. The easiest and most understandable way to do this is using a scale of 1-10 to rate your level of intensity based on how hard you feel you are working. Ten represents your maximal effort and one represents very-little, or no effort at all.

Eventually, as your body begins to adapt to your exercise program you will want to increase your intensity level. Always start slowly and gradually. Increase your exercise intensity over a relatively long period of time. Take small steps as you progress and do not try to do too much, too soon. Remember, "line upon line, precept upon precept, here a little and there a little" (2 Nephi 28:30).

Rest Time

The amount of time you rest between each set is very important if you want maximize the effects of your exercise program, especially since you are limited to only thirty-minutes of daily exercise time.

If your health and fitness goals are either to lose excess body fat or general fitness, your rest time between exercises should only be about one-minute. If you are exercising to increase muscle size, your rest time should be in the 1-2 minute range. If you are exercising to increase strength or power, your rest time between sets should be in the range of 2-5 minutes. To maximize your rest time, briefly stretch the muscles you just exercised between sets. This will help with flexibility and muscle recovery.

Recovery Time

Recovery is often the forgotten component in an exercise program. Optimal recovery time between exercise sessions is important to maximize your progress. During exercise your muscle tissue breaks down. It is during the recovery period between exercise sessions, rather than during the workout itself, that your muscles are allowed to rebuild. It is necessary to give the muscles in each movement pattern at least a day or two of recovery before exercising them again otherwise you run the risk of overtraining which could result in excess pain, discomfort, and even injury.

Likewise, you should also plan to significantly decrease your exercise intensity for about 5-7 days every six weeks, or more specifically, every 40 days. This is called a "recovery week" and its purpose is to give the body time to recover from the previous several weeks of hard work, allowing your body time to realize the progress you have made. As a general rule, you should not stop exercising altogether during recovery weeks, but rather, decrease the intensity and number of sets and reps you perform compared to what you have been doing.

In addition to a recovery week, every six-weeks, or 40 days, you should take an "active-rest" week (about 5-7 days) every twelfth week, or 120 days. This active-rest week will fall on the same regularly scheduled week as the recovery week. However, this week is different than the recovery week, because during this active-rest week, you will not just decrease your intensity and number of sets and reps, but you will participate in a completely different form of physical activity at a relatively low intensity (like playing basketball or some other sport instead of performing energy system and resistance training exercises).

The idea behind an active rest week is to give you time to perform other enjoyable, physical activities while getting away from the monotony of what you have been doing. Most importantly, this allows you to have a renewed vigor and focus when you return to your regular exercise program.

Personal Assistance

If you are not already doing so, get your companion involved in an exercise program with you. You might find it easier to maintain an exercise program if you are accountable to someone else. The two of you, together, can make sure you are exercising each day during the allotted exercise period. By partnering up with your companion during this time you will be able to offer support and encouragement to one another, in addition to assisting each other with some of the exercises.

The remaining elements of an exercise program, not discussed in this chapter, are performance-related and are covered in a companion guide to this book titled: *Missionary Fitness for Athletes*, available at www.missionaryfitness.com. This guide is for those missionaries who will be returning to athletic competition of any kind following their mission. It includes advanced exercise routines and information on a variety of topics specific to the missionary-athlete.

EXERCISE LOCATION

Locating a place to exercise while on your mission will take a bit of initiative and creativity on your part. In most situations, because of time and travel constraints, you will be limited to performing your exercises in, or around, your missionary apartment. However, you may find that you have a wealth of resources and locations available for exercising within a relatively short distance from your apartment where you can significantly increase the quality of your workouts.

Remember the benefits of fresh air and sunshine. Get outdoors and find a park, a playground, or even a jogging track at a local school or university near your apartment. Chances are you can find one of these nearby that has monkey bars, swings, and other recreational equipment that can be used to perform basic exercises. Parks often have an area or surface on which you can jog. A big benefit to exercising at a park or jogging track is they are usually open so if your companion does not want to exercise he can sit in the middle of the park or track and study while you exercise or jog nearby, staying within his view.

Differences in weather, air quality, altitude, and terrain must be considered when choosing a place to exercise. When exercising outdoors pay attention to any environmental concerns that may affect your health as you exercise. When exercising in high-altitudes, hot and/or humid climates reduce the intensity and duration of your workout until you have given your body plenty of time to adapt to the environmental conditions. For safety and health concerns you should avoid exercising along busy roads or highways where pollution levels are higher and where there is a significantly greater danger of getting injured.

When the weather or air-quality is poor consider exercising at an alternative location such as the gym at a local high school or university, the exercise room at a hotel or apartment complex in your area, or even at a nearby fitness center or health club. Creativity is the key to finding and making the most of what your mission and area have to offer.

Most places will understand your situation as a missionary and will be sympathetic to your health and fitness needs. They may allow you to exercise at their location for a reduced price or even for free. Ask if they have a clergy discount, or ask if you can provide some type of service during your weekly service hours in exchange for access to their facilities. Plus, you never know when these locations might produce missionary opportunities.

Remember, wherever you choose to exercise, you are still a missionary and must continue to obey all mission rules. You should never put exercise above your missionary work. It should never interfere with your missionary activities or your ability to perform your duties and responsibilities as a missionary. For obvious reasons you should avoid any location that plays music, has televisions, or magazines available during the time you will be there. Also, stay away from workout facilities where members of the opposite sex may be present at the same time. Always get approval from your mission president before exercising anywhere other than your missionary apartment.

SPECIAL CONSIDERATIONS

Most physical activity and exercise programs are considered beneficial because of their positive effects on overall general health. As you follow a regular exercise program and maintain a healthy diet you will be blessed to experience joy and happiness. However, the potential risk for injury and other health-related concerns exists with the addition of an exercise program and the increase in physical activity that accompanies missionary service.

The Missionary Fitness exercise and nutrition program has been specifically designed to help your body adapt quickly to new environments and stresses. By properly following the guidelines outlined in this book your body will begin the process of correcting muscular imbalances and postural weaknesses, significantly reducing and even eliminating common injuries and health concerns that plague missionaries.

Fortunately, the incidence and severity of exercise-related injuries and health concerns can also be reduced and eliminated by understanding the risks, taking preventative measures, and properly caring for them if they should arise. This section identifies and recommends proper preventative actions and treatments for a few of the more common missionary-related injuries and health concerns.

Asthma

Asthma is a chronic inflammation and narrowing of the airways, obstructing normal airflow to the lungs, resulting in labored breathing or shortness of breath. Asthma may be brought on by external factors that include contaminants in the air, such as smoke, pollution, dust, allergens, molds, animal dander, pollen, exposure to extreme temperatures, exercise, and stress. Symptoms may include coughing, wheezing, tightness or pain in the chest, prolonged shortness of breath, and extreme fatigue.

For alleviating symptoms of asthma and to prevent an asthma attack from occurring during exercise or intense physical activity precautions should be taken. These precautions include: exercising indoors, keeping the air-quality in your apartment as clean and dust-free as possible, taking asthma-related prescribed medications prior to exercise, warming-up and cooling-down sufficiently before and after any intense activity, avoiding physical exertion in extremely cold weather, when allergens are present, or when you have a respiratory infection. If you do experience an asthma attack while exercising, stop immediately and follow the appropriate action plan you should have established in advance with your health care provider.

Fatigue

Fatigue is a symptom of various other health concerns. Improper dietary habits, physical and/or emotional stress, hormone imbalances, infection, environmental factors, and any other stressors to the body can cause and emphasize fatigue. Typically, people reach for stimulants such as sugar, caffeine, and other substances to try and boost energy levels. This may cause more fatigue since the body has to exert additional energy, ridding itself of the unnatural stimulant.

Although it may seem detrimental to exercise, mild to moderate exercise like a walk outdoors or a basic exercise program such as the one outlined in this book will help the body gain more energy. Rest is obviously very important when the body is fatigued. This may include sleep, deep relaxation, and participating in meaningful leisure activities. For more on this read the "Resting from Your Labors" chapter.

Foot Problems

For many missionaries, the feet are the main method of transportation, so it is important you take good care of them. Unfortunately, because you are required to use them repeatedly, they are exposed to potential harm. The two most common foot problems missionaries experience are: blisters and ingrown toenails. Blisters are typically caused by friction from footwear that repeatedly rubs on the toes or heels of the foot. You can avoid blisters by reducing the amount of friction on your feet by wearing correctly-sized shoes, multiple pairs of socks, or by powdering your feet with a foot powder. If you do get a blister, leave it unbroken and avoid putting pressure on it or irritating it in any way. If the blister has already broken, keep it clean and dry with fresh bandages and antibiotic cream to protect it.

Ingrown toenails develop when the corner of the

toenail penetrates through the skin of the toe, damaging the underlying tissue, resulting in inflammation, pain, and sometimes infection. You can avoid ingrown toenails by properly caring for your feet. Trim your toenails regularly by cutting straight across the top of the nail. Never cut the sides or corners of the nail as this is where the ingrown toenail may develop. Wearing shoes that fit properly in length and width will also help prevent ingrown toenails.

If an ingrown toenail does develop, treat it by soaking the affected foot in lukewarm water several times a day. Epsom salt may be added to the water to help ease the inflammation and pain. After soaking it, thoroughly dry the foot and place a small piece of cotton underneath the corner of the nail to lift it up and away from the skin. Apply antibiotic cream and cover with a bandage.

When exercising with either of these foot conditions, avoid movements that put excess pressure or irritation on the injured area, allowing it time to heal and avoiding the risk of infection. Choose alternative exercises whenever possible to maintain consistency with your exercise program.

Hypoglycemia/Hyperglycemia

Hypoglycemia is a condition in which a person has low levels of glucose - or sugar - in their blood. This condition is usually related to an inadequate consumption of carbohydrates resulting in impaired brain function, light-headedness, irritability, constant fatigue, anxiety, lack of endurance or strength, trembles or shakes, hunger, heart palpitations, nervousness, and depression. To help alleviate the symptoms of hypoglycemia, eat six small meals a day and avoid consuming refined sugars and stimulants such as caffeine. If hypoglycemic reactions occur during exercise, stop immediately and eat or drink a simple carbohydrate like a piece of fruit, candy, or juice.

Hyperglycemia is a condition in which a person has excessive amounts of glucose circulating in their blood. This condition is most commonly caused by diabetes. If you suffer from this condition you should already be under medical supervision and have the necessary medication and knowledge to treat it.

Regular exercise and physical activity is an accepted and important therapy in the management of both hypoglycemia and hyperglycemia. People with these conditions are predisposed to many chronic diseases and health concerns that can be reduced by participating regularly in an exercise program. In addition, a healthy diet plays a significant role in properly managing the effects of these ailments.

Strains/Sprains

Strains refer to excessively stretching or tearing the muscle tissue or tendons and, in contrast, sprains refer to comparable damage to a ligament. Ankles and knees are the most common joints for this kind of damage to occur. This type of injury will cause limited movement, swelling, pain, and discoloration of the surrounding skin. If you experience a strain or sprain you should limit all movement in the affected area and follow the treatment plan affectionately known as R.I.C.E. Rest the injured area for at least 24 hours. This allows time for the body to manage the effects of the trauma while avoiding additional damage. Ice the area several times throughout the first two days and avoid taking hot bathes or applying heating pads. Ice lowers the temperature of the injured area reducing the breakdown of healthy cells and tissues. It can also reduce pain and swelling which accompany such injuries. Compress the area with an elastic bandage. Compression controls the swelling and prevents excess blood from accumulating in the damaged region. The support of such a wrap also decreases the occurrence of unnecessary movement. Elevate the affected limb above the level of the heart whenever possible. This will limit the swelling and help prevent fluids from pooling in the injured limb. By taking these measures you will allow your body to immediately begin the process of healing.

Do not return to full activity until the swelling and discoloration has significantly subsided in the wounded area. This does not mean, however, that you should avoid participating in physical activities while recovering. As with any injury or health concern you should still remain as active as possible by participating in alternative exercises that do not involve the injured muscle, joint, or limb.

Temperature-Related Health Problems

The human body is amazing at adapting to nearly any climate in the world. However, extended exposure to extreme temperatures can result in some serious health concerns. Heat-related illnesses are the most common of the temperature-related health problems precipitated by exercise. Heat-related illnesses are typically a function of several factors including the environment, intensity of physical activity, degree of exposure, hydration levels, type of clothing worn, and pre-existing physical condition. Following is a brief description of the three most serious conditions with their treatment:

Heat Cramps: Heat cramps can cause heavy perspiration and painful, tingling sensations throughout the arms, legs, and torso. If you experience this, remove yourself from the heat and find a cool place to rest. Loosen or remove any excess clothing and drink plenty of water to replenish lost fluids.

Heat Exhaustion: If heat cramps are not treated properly, they can quickly turn into heat exhaustion. Heat exhaustion causes intense thirst, dizziness, rapid heart rate, muscle cramps, nausea, vomiting, fatigue, and mental confusion. To treat this condition, follow the same guidelines for treating heat cramps. Additionally, try to keep your body temperature down by cooling off with a fan, ice, cold bathes, or applying moist, cool towels to your body.

Heat Stroke: Heat stroke is a life-threatening emergency condition. It is differentiated from heat exhaustion in that the body temperature rises above 105 degrees Fahrenheit. Convulsions, confusion, unconsciousness, lack of perspiration, and rapid heart rate are also definitive symptoms. Follow the same procedures for treating heat exhaustion and promptly obtain assistance from emergency medical personnel.

Heat illnesses may be prevented by maintaining adequate levels of hydration and avoiding exercise and increased physical activity in extremely hot or humid environments.

If other, more serious, injuries or health concerns arise, or current conditions persist for an unreasonable amount of time then you should discuss them with your mission president. Talk with him if you have any questions or concerns about any health or medical-related problems. All medical and health care should be coordinated through your mission president. He will refer you to the appropriate health and medical professionals to evaluate, diagnose, and treat any condition you may have.

FIT FOR SERVICE, PART II
Putting It All Together

Incorporating an exercise program into your everyday mission life is easier than you might think. However, putting together an effective exercise program is not a simple procedure. Fortunately, the information provided in this chapter will take the guesswork out of it by assimilating all of the information from the previous chapter and integrating it into a useful exercise program that will prepare you for service. The following exercise program contains everything you need to transform your body and spirit while you prepare for and serve your mission. It has been designed to be simple, yet intense and to be practical, yet effective. It has been designed for the unique lifestyle of a full-time missionary.

All of the exercises demonstrated in this exercise program use bodyweight as the primary form of resistance. If you have access to other methods of resistance or exercise equipment then please refer to the companion book to this book titled: *Additional Exercises for Missionary Fitness*, available at www.missionaryfitness.com.

WARMING-UP TO A GREAT WORKOUT – DYNAMIC STRETCHING

Warming-up for energy system training and resistance training are slightly different. Prior to performing energy system training you should warm-up by performing the exercise you plan to do for the workout (for example; walking, jogging, bike riding, stair climbing, or rope jumping, etc.) at a low-intensity for a 3-5 minutes, or until you begin to sweat.

Before beginning resistance training you should warm-up by performing dynamic stretches. Dynamic stretching is a great tool to bridge the gap between inactivity and your resistance training activity, while saving time and preparing you physically and mentally for the workout to come.

Dynamic stretches should include 5-10 repetitions of each stretch, gradually increasing both tempo and range of motion when appropriate. The idea is to start slow and shallow and progress by going faster and further. For each stretch, you should only go to the point where you begin to feel tension on the targeted muscle and no more. The entire dynamic stretching sequence should only take about 3-5 minutes at the beginning of resistance training.

Dynamic Stretching Warm-up: Perform at the beginning of resistance training days.

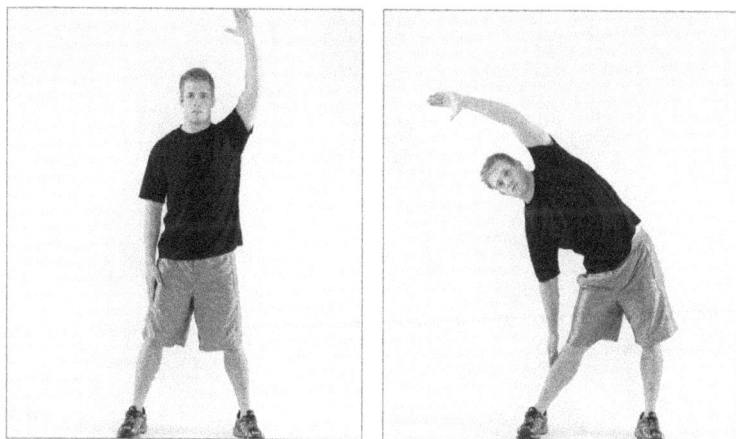

Side Bends: Stand with your feet slightly wider than hip-width apart and one arm extended straight above your head. Place the opposite arm straight down at your side. Slowly bend to the side while running your hand down your leg. Go until you feel a good stretch in your side. Return to the starting position and repeat 5-10 times. Switch sides and perform this exercise on the other side 5-10 times.

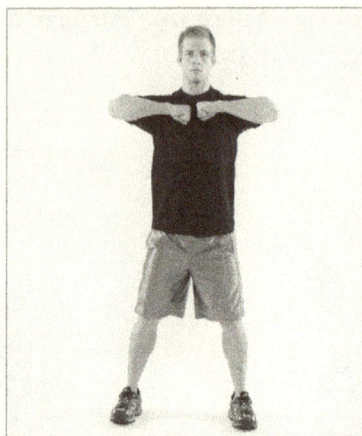

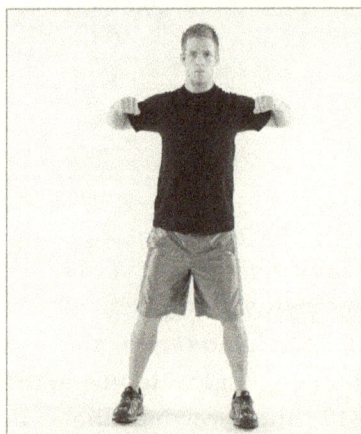

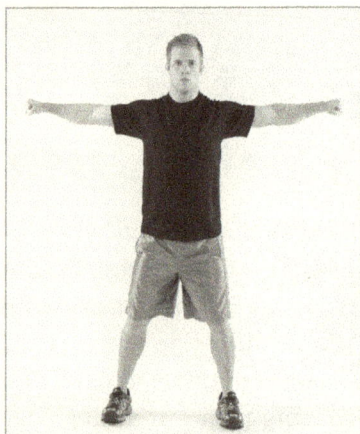

Arms Horizontal: Raise both arms in front of you making a fist with each hand. Then bend your elbows outward until the knuckles of each hand are touching in front of your chest. Next, extend both arms out to the side, so your elbows are going toward your back opening your arms until they are completely straight and horizontal to the floor. Return to the starting position. Perform 5-10 repetitions.

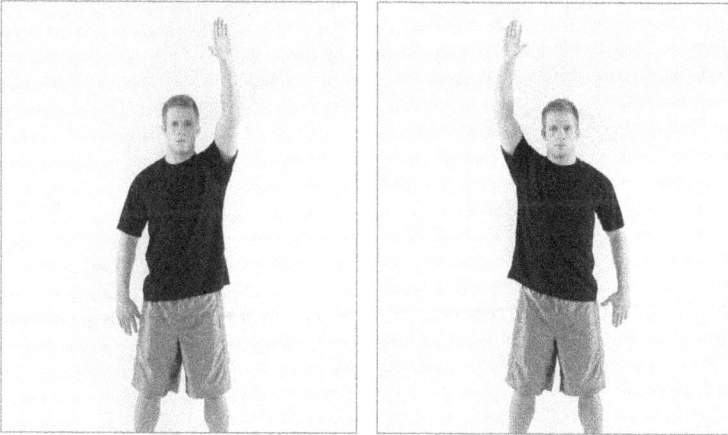

Arms Vertical: Start by raising one arm up in front of you into a vertical position while the other arm remains down and slightly behind your torso. Alternate this movement by raising the other arm vertically as you lower the extended arm back down until your forearm extends slightly behind your torso. Increase the speed of this movement with each repetition. Repeat 5-10 times with each arm.

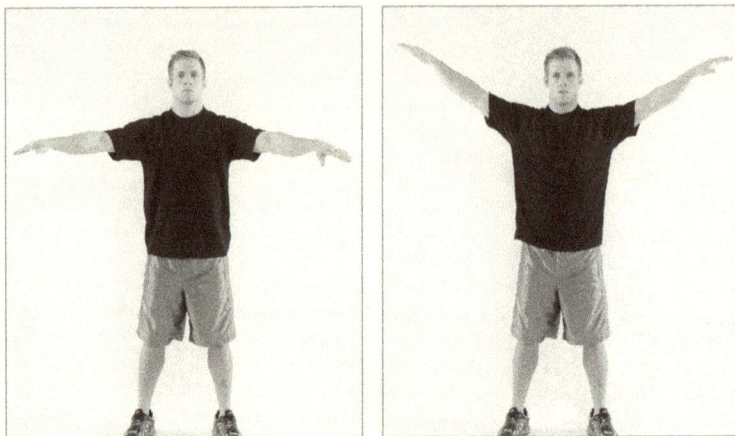

Arm Circles: With your arms straight out to your sides in a horizontal position, rotate them forward in small circles gradually increasing the diameter of the circles with each repetition. Switch directions and rotate your arms backwards in small circles gradually increasing to larger circles with each repetition. Repeat 5-10 times for each direction.

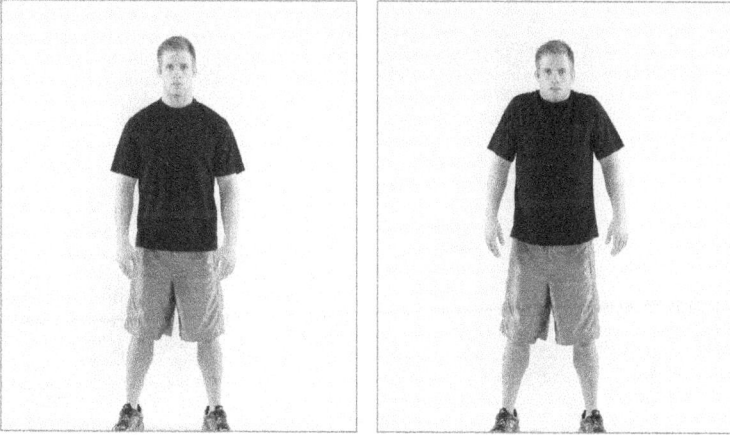

Shoulder Shrugs: Keeping your arms straight down at your side, elevate your shoulders up as high as possible. Hold this position for a second, and then let them down. Repeat 5-10 times.

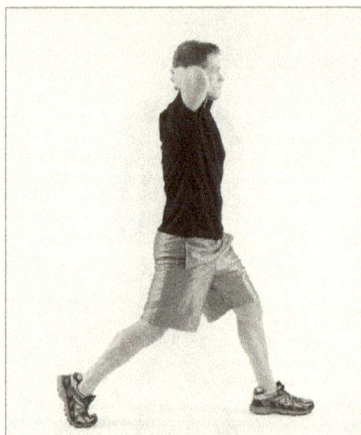

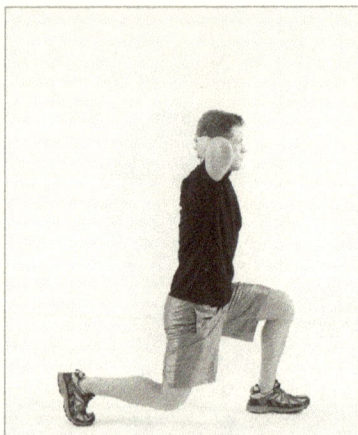

Split Squats: Stand with one leg 3 to 4 feet in front of the other, with your toes pointed forward. Keep your torso erect. Clasp your hands behind your head. Bend both knees to lower your body straight down until your back knee is a few inches off the floor and your front leg is bent at a 90-degree angle (the thigh parallel to the floor and the lower leg perpendicular to the floor). Return to the starting position and repeat 5-10 times on both legs.

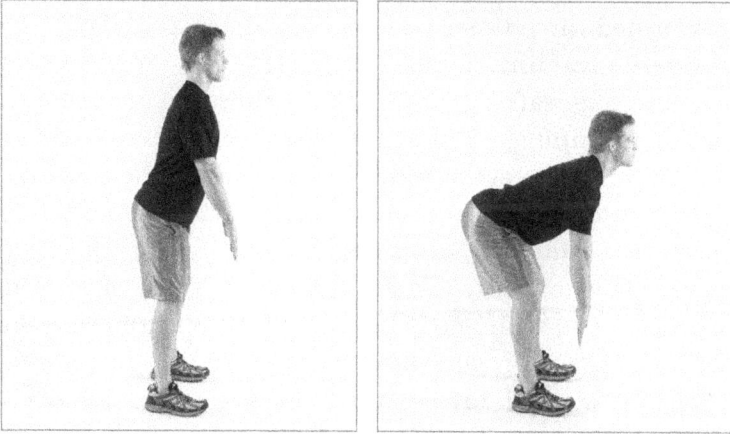

Toe Touches: With your feet slightly wider than hip-width apart and your knees slightly bent, bend over at your waist and touch your toes. Return to the starting position and repeat 5-10 times.

If you have followed this dynamic stretching warm-up routine correctly, you should feel warm, strong, loose, and enthusiastic about beginning your workout.

SERVE WITH ALL YOUR HEART – ENERGY SYSTEM TRAINING

Energy system training should last 20 to 25 minutes, not including the warm-up and cool-down, and should be performed three times per week on alternating days with resistance training. First, select an energy system training exercise like walking, jogging, bike riding, stair climbing, or rope jumping. You should vary your energy system training exercise every session, if possible, for best results.

After selecting the exercise, start with a three to five-minute, low-intensity warm-up, or until you break a light sweat. Low-intensity would be a level of three or four on a scale of 1-10 with one being the easiest and 10 being the most intense effort you could ever put forth.

Now, after breaking a light sweat you are ready to begin the actual workout. Begin by increasing your intensity to a level of eight or nine. At this level you will perform the exercise for 15 seconds followed by a decrease in intensity to a moderate level, about a six or seven, for 30 seconds. Repeat this pattern of alternating between high-intensity and moderate-intensity for 20 to 25 minutes. After completing this, lower your intensity to a level of a three or four for a cool-down of approximately three-minutes.

When the intervals of 15 seconds at high-intensity and 30 seconds at moderate-intensity become too easy, you can increase both interval times in increments of 15 seconds while still maintaining the pattern above. By increasing the interval times in this manner there comes a point of diminishing returns where the interval times become too much. These interval times will be different for everyone so proceed with caution and stay under them once you determine what they are for yourself.

Another way of challenging yourself is to decrease the time between the high-intensity and moderate-intensity exercises so they match. For example, perform at a high-intensity for 30 seconds and a moderate-intensity for 30 seconds or 45 seconds of high-intensity followed by 45 seconds of moderate-intensity. Feel free to experiment and adjust the high-intensity to moderate-intensity ratios according to your own level of health and fitness. However, remember to proceed with caution and do not push so hard that you feel dizzy, faint, nauseous, or that you are unable to continue for the duration of the training session.

If you are trying to lose excess body-fat then your energy system training should be performed first thing in the morning on an empty stomach. This way you will burn body-fat as fuel instead of food. If you are not trying to lose excess body fat and your goal is to increase muscle mass, you should perform your energy system training after eating a simple meal high in carbohydrates and moderately-high in protein.

SERVE WITH ALL YOUR STRENGTH – RESISTANCE TRAINING

Resistance training should last 20 to 25 minutes and be performed three times per week on alternating days with energy system training. Using the information in the previous chapter, select the appropriate sets, reps, and rest time to be used based on your individual health needs and fitness goals. Before you begin your resistance training make sure you have already performed an adequate warm-up using dynamic stretches.

TOTAL-BODY RESISTANCE TRAINING WORKOUT A:

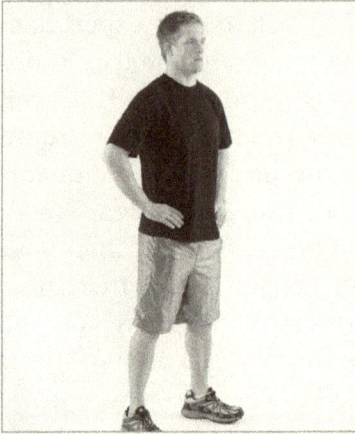

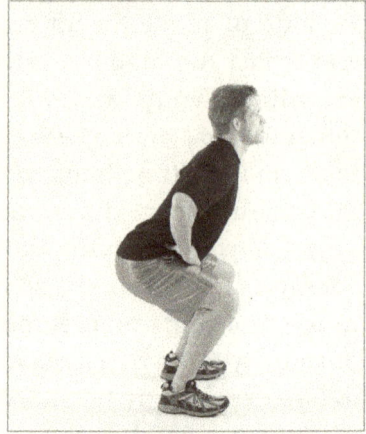

A1: Quad-Dominant Movement – Squat:

Stand with your feet hip-width apart with a slight bend in your knees. Keeping all of your weight on your heels and bending at your knees, sit back like you are sitting in a chair. While keeping your knees behind the plane of your toes throughout the entire range of motion sit back or squat until your upper thighs are parallel to the ground (or as far down as you feel comfortable while maintaining proper form). Pause, and then push yourself back up to the starting position. For a greater challenge, increase the amount of resistance by adding weight.

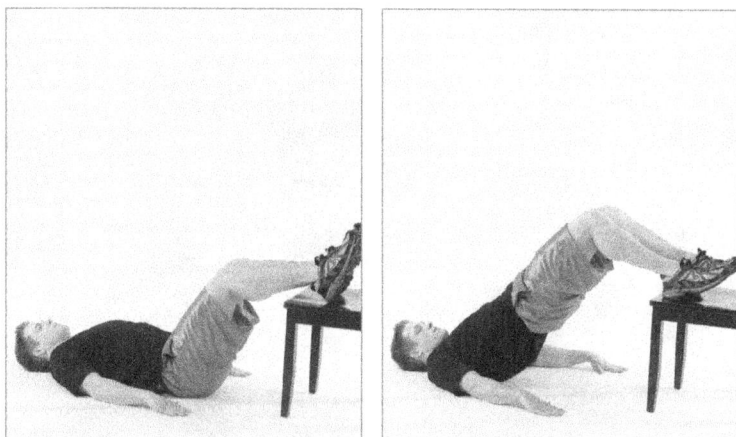

A2: Hip-Dominant Movement –
Lying Hip Extension:

Lie on the floor with your arms at your sides and both heels up on a chair or bench, with your knees bent. Drive your heels down into the seat of the chair to lift your hips up until your body forms a straight line from your knees to your shoulders. Pause, and return to the starting position. For a greater challenge, straighten one leg and hold it over your hip so you are only using one leg to lift your hips up. For an even greater challenge try doing this exercise using only one leg at a time.

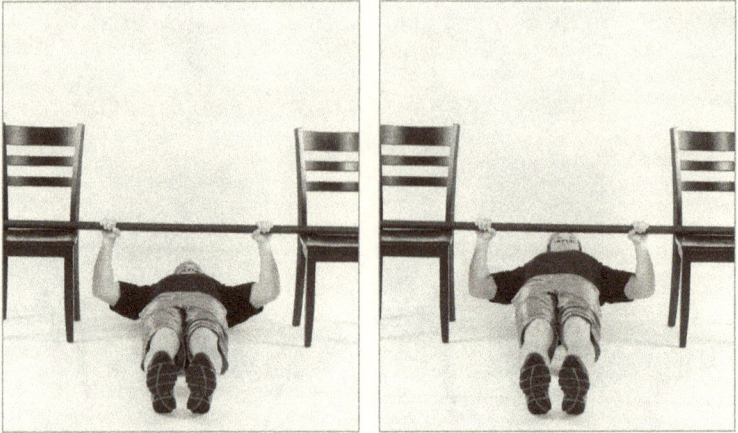

B1: Horizontal Pulling Movement – Lying Back Row:

Place a sturdy broomstick or something similar between two chairs spread about three or four feet apart. Lie down under the bar so it is directly over your chest. Grab it with an overhand; slightly wider than shoulder-width-apart grip. Lift your body off the floor so only the back of your heels remain on the floor. Be sure to hold your body in a straight line from your head to your heels. At the top of the movement, pinch your shoulder blades together as you pull your chest up as close as possible to the bar. For a greater challenge, rest your feet on a raised surface such as a chair or a bench.

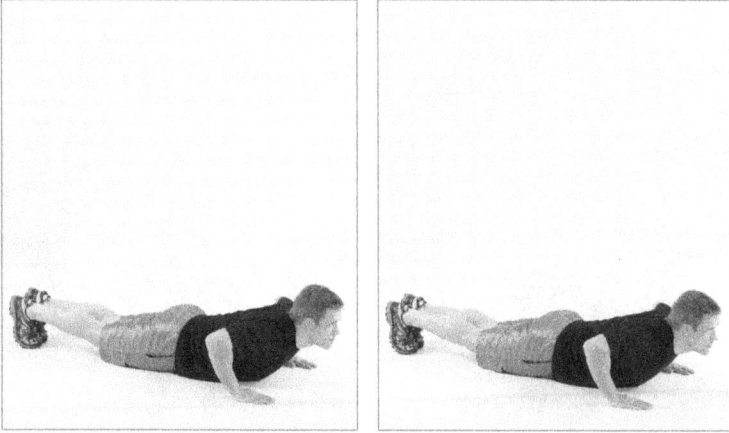

B2: Horizontal Pushing Movement – Pushup:
Position your hands slightly wider than shoulder-width apart, palms flat on the floor and support your body with your hands and the balls of your feet. Straighten your arms without locking your elbows. Lower your torso until your chest is about an inch off the floor. Push yourself back to the starting position. For a greater challenge, put one foot on top of the other, put both feet up on a raised surface, or place your hands closer or wider apart.

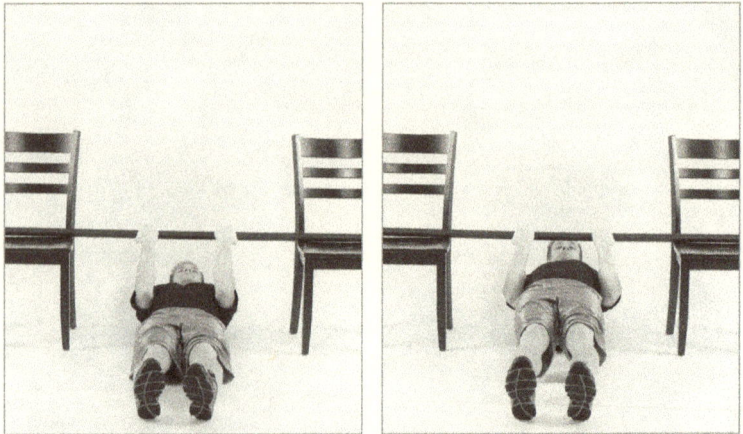

C1: Arm Pulling Movement – Lying Biceps Curl:
Place a sturdy broomstick or something similar between two chairs spread about three or four feet apart. Lie down under the bar so it is directly over your chest. Grab it with an underhand; slightly narrower than shoulder-width-apart grip. Lift your body off the floor so only the back of your heels remain on the floor. Be sure to hold your body in a straight line from your head to your heels. Pull your body up by curling your arms until your chest is as close as possible to the bar. For a greater challenge, rest your feet on a raised surface such as a chair or a bench.

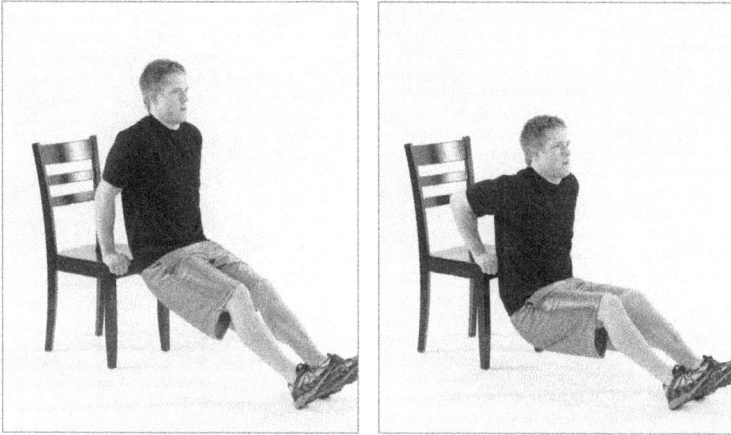

C2: Arm Pushing Movement – Chair Dip:

Hold on to the edge of a sturdy chair behind you, with your knees bent and your feet flat on the floor. Keep your back arched and close to the chair. Slowly lower your body until the back of your upper arms are parallel to the floor. Your torso should remain straight throughout the entire range of motion. Pause for a second, and press back up to the starting position. To make this exercise more challenging, straighten your legs out in front of you or elevate your feet on a raised surface.

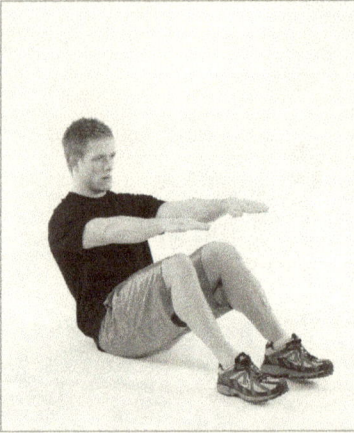

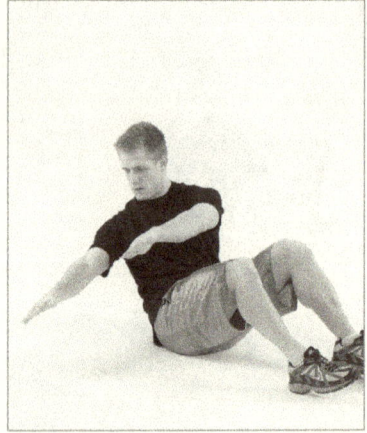

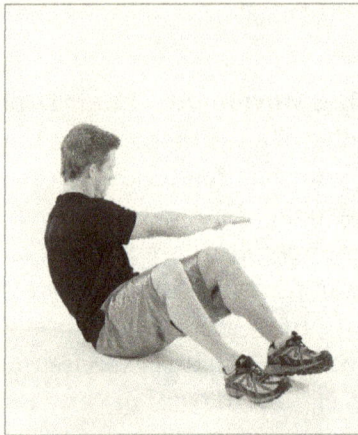

D1: Core Rotational Movement – Abdominal Twist:

Sit on the ground with your torso at a 45-degree angle to the floor (as if you are halfway through a sit-up) with your arms stretched directly out in front of you. Bend your knees and keep your feet free (not anchored by anything). While maintaining this torso angle, rotate as far as possible to one side and then, without pausing, rotate to the other side.

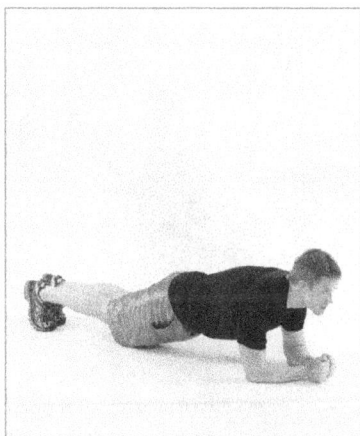

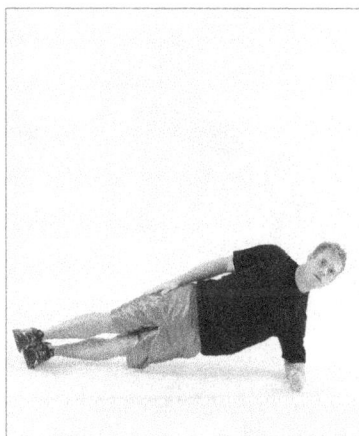

D2: Core Stabilization Movement – Front/Side Plank:

Get into a modified pushup position by supporting your weight on your forearms and toes. Your body should form a straight line from your head to your heels (do not let your back sag). Pull your abs in as far as you can and hold this position for 20 to 60 seconds. Rotate to one side and support your weight with your forearm and the outside edge of your foot. Your body should form a straight line from your head to your ankles. Pull your abs in as far as you can, hold this position for 20 to 60 seconds. Repeat on the other side for 20 to 60 seconds. Rest the appropriate time period for your goal, and repeat.

TOTAL-BODY RESISTANCE TRAINING WORKOUT B:

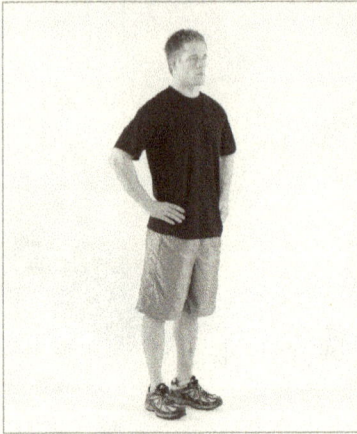

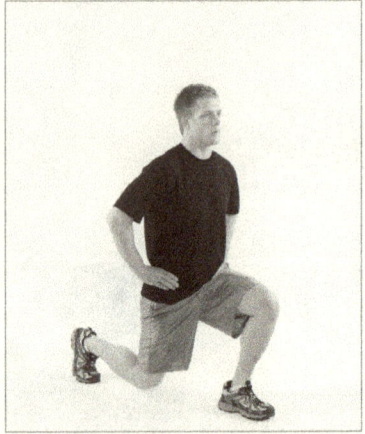

A1: Quad-Dominant Movement – Lunge:

Stand with your feet hip-width apart and your hands on your hips. Take a long step forward so your front foot lands two to three feet in front of you, and lower your body until the top of your front thigh is parallel to the floor. Your forward knee should be directly over your ankle and should never extend in front of your toes. Now, explosively push yourself back to the starting position. For an even greater challenge try the single-leg squat.

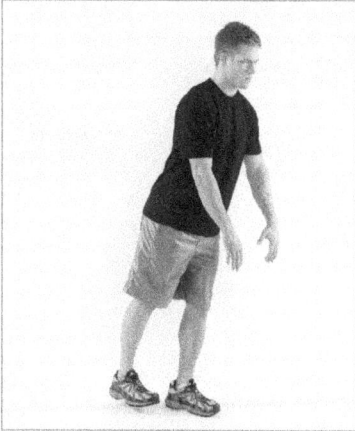

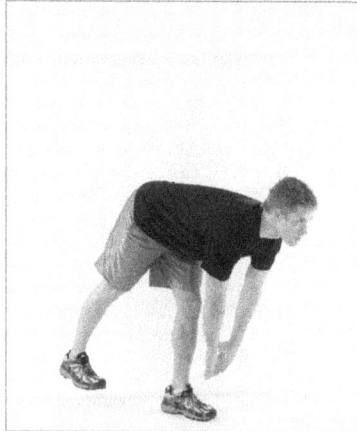

A2: Hip-Dominant Movement –
Single, Straight-Leg Deadlift:

Stand with your feet hip-width apart, knees slightly bent, abdominals tucked in, shoulders pulled back, and arms at your sides. Lift one foot an inch or two off the floor. Bending at the hips, lower your torso until it is as close to parallel to the floor as you can get without rounding your back. Pause, and push through your heel to go back up.

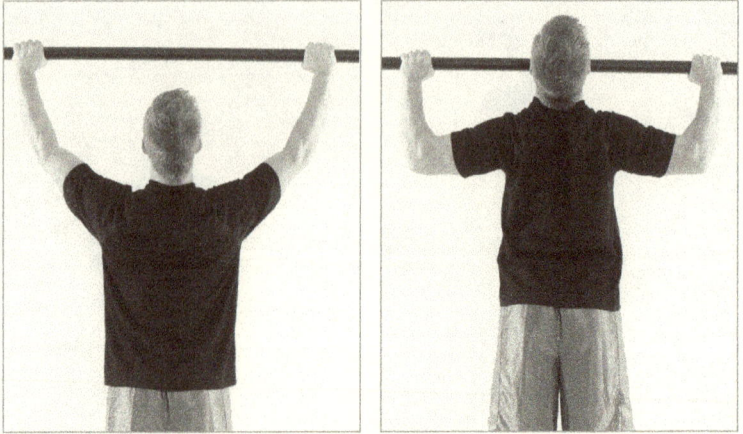

B1: Vertical Pulling Movement – Pull Up:

Grab a pull-up bar, or any other sturdy overhead structure, with an overhand, shoulder-width apart grip, and hang with your elbows slightly bent. Pull your body up until your chin is slightly above the bar, hold for a second or two. Finish by lowering your body under control back to the starting position. To increase the difficulty use a wider grip or wear a backpack full of heavy books.

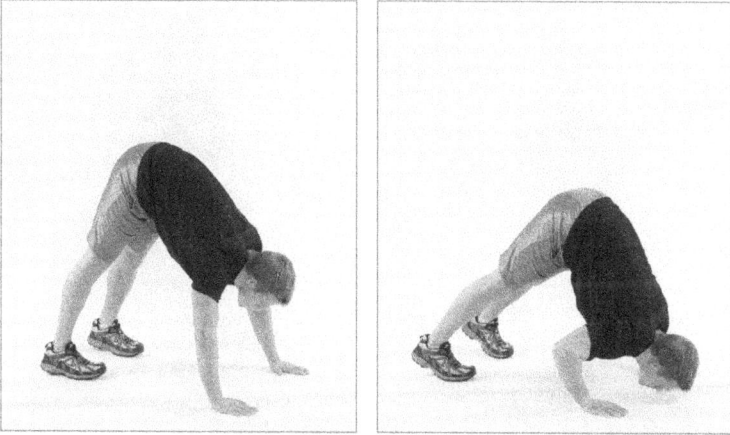

B2: Vertical Pushing Movement – Pike Pushup:

Get into the standard pushup position with your hands about shoulder-width apart. Walk your feet forward until they are 2-3 feet behind your hands and your hips are sticking up in the air. Lean all of your bodyweight over your shoulders. Keep your legs straight as you bend your arms and bring your face to the floor. Push back up to the starting position. To make this movement more challenging, perform a handstand pushup against a wall.

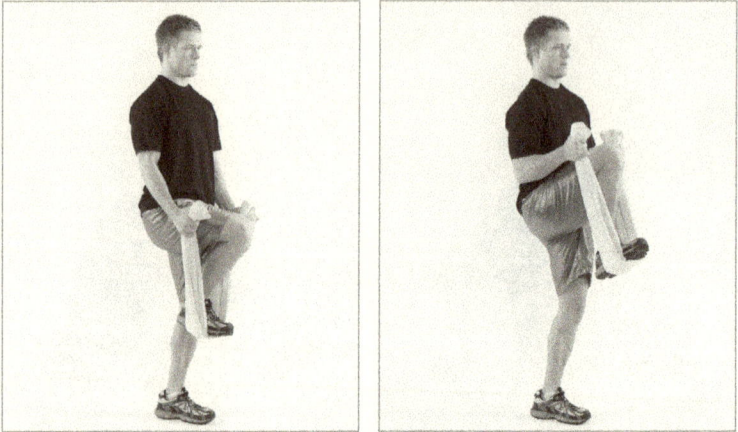

C1: Arm Pulling Movement – Towel Curl:

Fold a large bath towel lengthwise a few times and hold it at either end, with your palms facing each other, as you stand with your back against a wall. Move your feet out about a foot in front of you, and place one of them in the middle of the towel. Start with both knees slightly bent. With your arms straight down, curl your arms upward toward your shoulders while using your foot to resist the movement. Pause at the top and use your arms to resist your leg's attempt to push the towel back down to the floor. Return to the starting position and repeat.

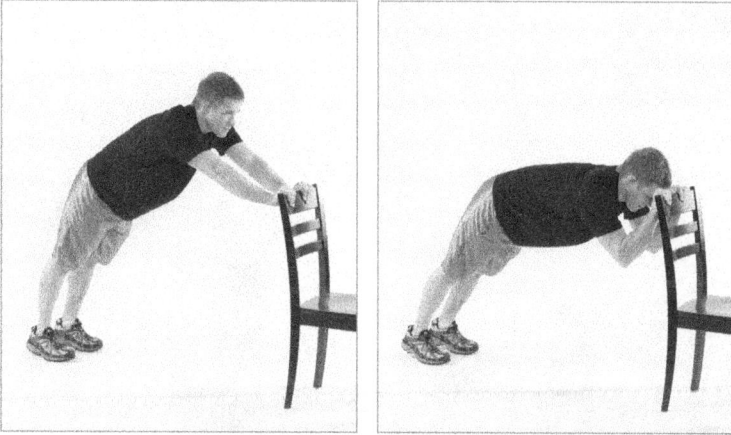

C2: Arm Pushing Movement – Triceps Extension:
Using the back of a chair, a stool, or table about waist height, grasp the edge with your hands, shoulder-width apart. Lock your elbows out to support your weight, move your feet back until you are in a semi-pushup position. Bend your elbows and lower your body so your head goes below the edge of the stool or table as much as possible. Pause, then press forward with your arms and raise yourself back to the starting position. To increase the difficulty, simply use a chair or other sturdy structure that is lower than waist height.

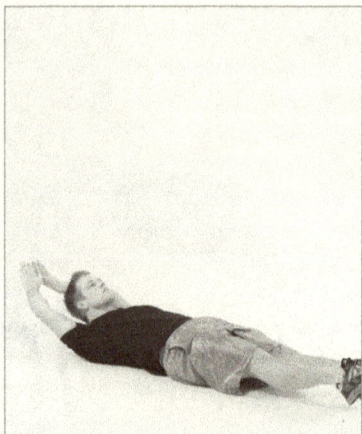

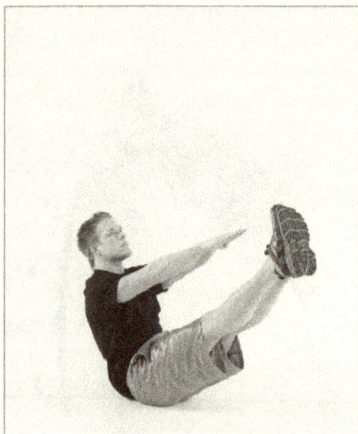

D1: Trunk/Hip Flexion Movement – Abdominal V-Sit Crunch:

Lie on your back, arms extended behind head and legs straight our in front of you. Raise both arms and legs towards each other, keeping legs as straight as possible and back flat. Touch your toes, shins, or whatever you can comfortably reach. Lower your body down using a controlled movement without letting your feet or hands touch the floor.

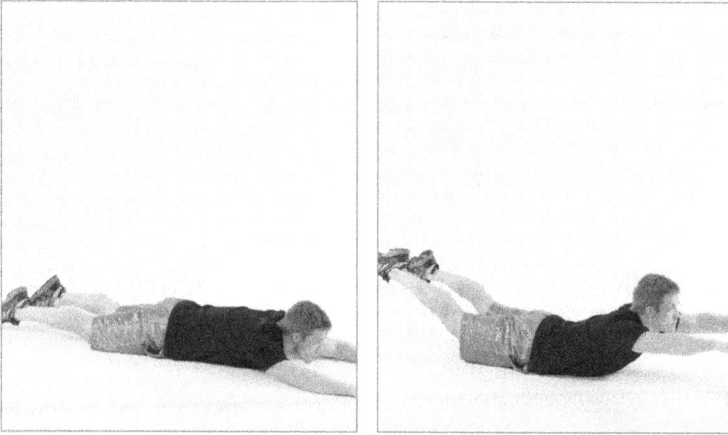

D2: Trunk/Hip Extension Movement – Lying Back Extension:

Lie facedown on the ground with your legs straight and your arms stretched out in front of you, with your hands on the floor. Lift your arms, head, chest, and legs off the floor simultaneously. Hold this position for 3-5 seconds, keeping your head and neck at the same height as your shoulders throughout the movement. Return to the starting position and repeat.

There are a couple things to consider when performing the exercises illustrated above: Pay close attention to proper breathing methods. Inhale as you begin each exercise, and exhale as you perform the movement. Never hold your breath during the exercises. In order to promote flexibility, ensure safety, and receive the maximum benefit each exercise should be performed using proper form throughout the complete range of motion. Never cheat yourself by failing to complete the entire movement. You will miss out on achieving greater success if you do.

For additional exercises and more advanced variations of these exercises check out the companion guide to this book titled: *Additional Exercises for Missionary Fitness* available at www.missionaryfitness.com.

COOLING-DOWN FROM A GREAT WORKOUT – STATIC STRETCHING

Performing a cool-down from your energy system training has already been discussed and is pretty straight-forward. Cooling-down from your resistance training involves static stretching and should take about three to five minutes to complete.

While the stretches given below are quite thorough, they do not target every single muscle group. This program is only the beginning. From there you can learn variations and techniques to individualize your flexibility training depending on your individual health needs and fitness goals. Here are some stretches to get you started:

Static Stretching Cool-down: Perform at the end of resistance training.

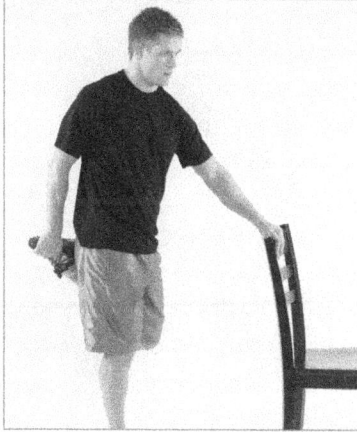

Quadriceps: To assist with balance grab an object in front of you and bend one of your knees. With the opposite hand, grab your foot and pull it toward your buttocks until you feel a mild stretch in the front of your thigh. Hold for 20 seconds, switch legs, and repeat. Make sure to keep your chest up and do not to let your back arch while performing this stretch.

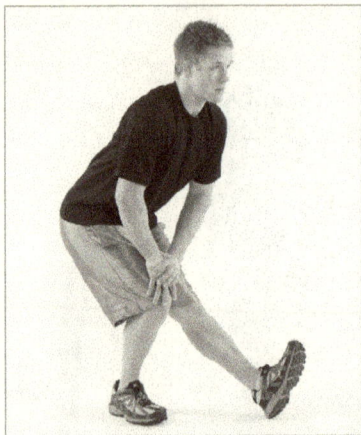

Hamstrings: Stand up straight with your chest held high and extend one foot out in front of you with your heel down and toe up. Bend the knee of the opposite leg and rest both hands on its upper thigh, push your buttocks back until you feel a mild stretch in your hamstrings (the back of your upper-leg). Make sure to keep an arch in your lower-back throughout the stretch. Hold for 20 seconds, switch legs, and repeat as often as necessary.

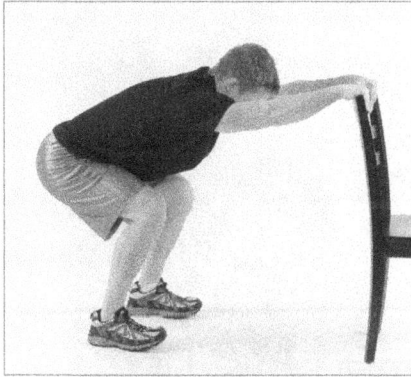

Back: Stand up straight with your chest held high and your hands on something stable just above waist height. From the starting position, push the buttocks back until you feel a mild stretch along the sides of your back. Hold for 20 seconds and repeat as necessary. This can also be done one arm at a time if you have one side that is significantly tighter than the other.

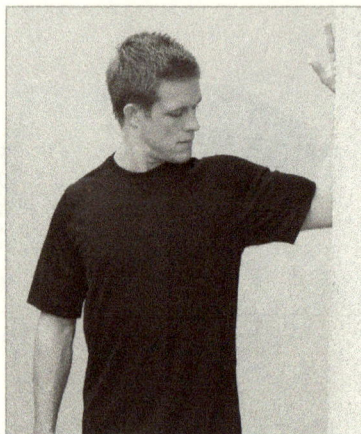

Chest: Using a doorway or post, bend your arm to 90-degrees and place the lower portion of your arm and hand along the length of the doorway. From this starting position, twist your hips in the opposite direction until you feel a mild stretch in your chest. Hold for 20 seconds, switch arms, and repeat.

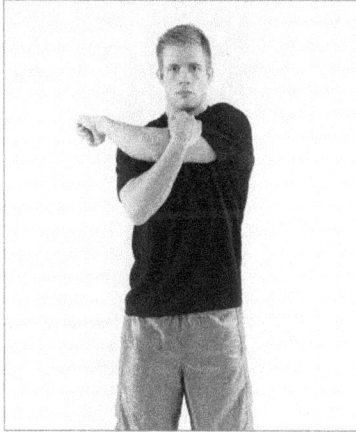

Shoulders: In a standing position, use one arm to pull the elbow of the opposite arm horizontally straight across your chest until you feel a mild stretch in your shoulder. Hold for 20 seconds and repeat on the other side.

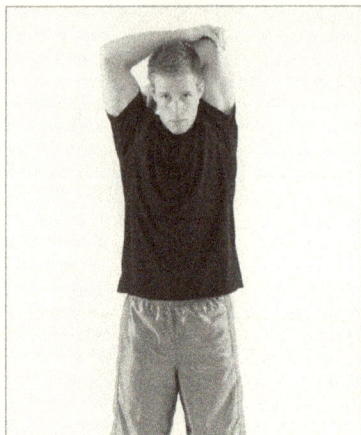

Triceps: In a standing position, flex your shoulder and bend your elbow to a point where your elbow is pointing straight up toward the ceiling. From there, using the opposite arm pull your elbow even farther back behind your head until you feel a mild stretch in the back of your upper arm. Hold for 20 seconds and repeat on the opposite side.

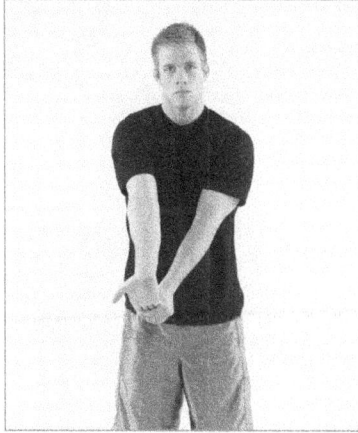

Biceps: In a standing position, extend one of your arms straight out in front of you with your palm facing up. With your opposite hand pull the other hand down until you feel a slight stretch in your biceps. Hold for 20 seconds and repeat on the opposite side.

Although every missionary will experience positive results from following this program, please realize that no single program will solve all the unique needs of every individual. This program is a general physical fitness program and should be used only as a guide. It is designed to easily be adapted to fit your individual health needs and fitness goals. If you are looking for something more specific you can visit www.missionaryfitness.com for additional exercise and nutrition resources.

SECTION III:

ENDURING
TO THE END

RESTING FROM YOUR LABORS

As a missionary, your labors are physically, spiritually, mentally, and emotionally demanding, sapping your energy, and leaving you tired and worn-out. The spirit can only sustain you for so long before physical exhaustion takes its toll and leaves you unable to perform the labors you are called to. Fortunately, the Lord has given clear instructions that we should not labor more than we have strength and that we need to rest from our labors (see D&C 10:4 and 59:10). By not resting adequately, you run the risk of getting sick or developing other health concerns, which may compromise your ability to serve as a missionary. If you are serious about becoming the best missionary you can, then you need to restore this lost energy each and every day by getting sufficient rest.

Resting from your labors and getting sufficient rest is not just about sleeping at night. It also includes establishing good sleeping habits, resting one day out of every seven, and recovering from physical exercise.

LIE DOWN UNTO THE LORD

Sleep is an essential part of life. Approximately one-third of your lifetime will be devoted to sleep. Disregarding the importance of it can lead to harmful consequences in your ability to serve. Each and every night after a long day of missionary work, the body and spirit are exhausted and need to be renewed. The physical and spiritual renewal process can only occur through sufficient amounts of quality sleep each night. The quality and amount of sleep you receive will directly affect your ability to perform as a missionary and your ability to handle the stress and pressures related to missionary life.

Surely Alma knew the importance of obtaining sufficient sleep when he said to his son Helaman, "Yea, when thou liest down at night lie down unto the Lord" (Alma 37:37). Alma was not just simply telling Helaman to say his prayers at night. Lying down unto the Lord means much more than just saying your prayers before bedtime. It also means that you should handover to the Lord all of the worries and concerns afflicting you. In this way your body, mind, and spirit can rest easily and peacefully during the night. This is not always easy to do, especially when the eternal salvation of souls rest on your shoulders. However, it is important that you learn how to do this to ensure you get the highest quality of sleep each night because it is only during sleep that several vital physiological processes can take place.

When the body is sleeping, it is free to restore damaged cells, repair injured organs, and renew wounded tissues. The mind uses this time to organize and integrate new information and sort out feelings and emotions. The spirit uses this time to receive inspiration and insight in finding solutions to pressing concerns. When these important processes are not allowed to occur due to inadequate sleep side effects begin to occur. Some of these side effects include irritability, nervousness, anxiety, weakened immune system function, weight gain, depression, and impaired ability to focus. Overall, the quality of your mission and your life is negatively affected by not getting sufficient, quality sleep.

The Lord has given clear instruction on what constitutes a sufficient amount of sleep when He said, "...cease to sleep longer than is needful; retire to thy bed early, that ye may not be weary; arise early, that your bodies and your minds may be invigorated" (D&C 88:124). Note that this scripture does not say you should get exactly eight hours of sleep, or exactly six hours, or even ten hours of sleep each night. It simply says to retire early and arise early. Everyone is different and so every person's sleep requirements differ slightly. Perhaps this is why the Lord did not stipulate an exact amount of time for sleep. However, most experts agree that adults need about seven to eight hours of sleep each night to ensure good health and sufficient energy.

It is not uncommon for missionaries to struggle with falling asleep at bedtime, even after a long day of hard work or to struggle with arising early, even after a long night of sleep. As a result, you may wake up when the alarm clock goes off and feel like you hardly received any sleep at all. Often the reason you do not feel well-rested in the morning may be related more to your waking hours. Stress, anxiety, fear, lack of physical activity, and poor nutritional habits can all negatively affect sleep patterns and cause sleep-related trouble.

Ensuring a good night sleep starts long before the lights go out. In fact, what you do during the day can do more for your sleep than anything else. Begin by making your sleep environment – your bedroom – as comfortable as possible. Sleep in a room that has good air circulation. Eliminate stale air by opening the windows at night, using a circulation fan, or keeping live plants in the room. Keep the room temperature regular and constant, on the cool side, about 65 degrees Fahrenheit. Sleep on a mattress that offers good support, using bedding that is clean and comfortable. Eliminate as much light and noise as possible in your bedroom. One way to eliminate noise is to drown it out with "white noise" from a fan, a trickling water fountain, or a bedside audio device that provides nature sounds. Put your alarm clock where you can not easily see it. If you happen to wake-up in the middle of the night you may not want to know what time it is, especially when it feels like you have slept for several hours but, in reality, it has been much less than what you thought. This can be very frustrating and can make it even more difficult for you to fall back to sleep.

Establish a routine you can follow consistently every night before going to bed. An established routine will help you relax and let your body know it is time to sleep. This routine should start about 20 or 30 minutes before your scheduled bedtime. It may include reading from the scriptures, writing in your journal, pondering, listening to peaceful music, taking a warm bath or shower, or any other activity you find relaxing. This should be a time to unwind and relax, not a time to worry about all the things you still need to do before going to bed or the things you need to do the next day.

Avoid eating or drinking very much within an hour or so of bedtime. Too much fluid at night may cause you to wake-up in the middle of the night to use the bathroom. Too much food may make you uncomfortable as you lie down, making it difficult to sleep. Do not overexert yourself physically at night because it can give you a renewal of energy, keeping you awake when you should be sleeping. Limit the amount of mental stimulation you get at night. This may cause you to think excessively, keeping you awake.

Something you might find helpful is to keep a

record of your sleeping habits. A recorded daily account of your sleeping habits can help you recognize certain patterns and behaviors that contribute to, or prevent you from getting adequate amounts of quality sleep each night. You can record the time you went to sleep, the time you woke-up, how many times you awoke, if any, during the night, the total number of hours you slept, the food you ate, and activities you did just before going to bed.

Look back at this information to figure out what behaviors promoted certain feelings. Repeat the effective behaviors that resulted in restful sleep and renewed energy and do away with the behaviors that resulted in poor sleep and little energy. These notes can be documented in your weekly planner or in the *Missionary Fitness Journal*, available free at www.missionaryfitness.com. Here are some additional suggestions to help you get the sleep you need:

- Get at least thirty-minutes of physical exercise each day and increase your level of physical activity throughout the day

- Eat good-quality, natural foods

- Avoid taking naps during the day – this is a real temptation for missionaries, especially at lunch time

- On occasion, when you need a nap in order to get you through the day, keep it short, limiting it to no more than 20 or 30 minutes

- Get plenty of fresh air and sunlight during the day, keeping your body's natural clock in-sync by regulating the sleep hormone, melatonin

A DAY...OR TWO OF REST

God has given everyone a special day to rest. This day is known as the Sabbath Day. In addition to this day of rest, God has given missionaries another special day for rest and temporal preparations. This day is known as Preparation Day or more affectionately referred to as P-Day. Each of these days serve a unique purpose and function in the life of full-time missionaries.

Sabbath Day

The scriptures are clear with the command to rest one day in every seven. "Six days shalt though labour, and do all thy work: But the seventh day is the sabbath of the Lord thy God; in it thou shalt not do any work" (Exodus 20:9-10). God created this day of rest and gave it to His children as a gift. Even God Himself, honors the eternal law of rest as demonstrated in Genesis, "And on the seventh day God ended his work which he had made; and he rested on the seventh day from all his work which he had made" (Genesis 2:2). The physical body uses this day of rest to allow it time to repair, renew, and recover while the spirit is free to grow closer to God.

For most faithful members of the Church, Sunday is in fact, a day of rest. However, for missionaries, Sunday is typically one of the busiest days of the week. In addition to your regular proselyting responsibilities, you will spend most Sundays attending meetings, perhaps even conducting, teaching, or presenting at these meetings, calling investigators, arranging rides to get your investigators to church, preparing for baptisms, scheduling appointments, visiting members, preparing and passing the sacrament, and any other responsibilities or duties you have that are unique to your mission. Unfortunately, because of this, it is difficult, if not impossible, for Sunday to be enjoyed by missionaries as a complete day of rest.

Perhaps this is why God has inspired the leaders of the Church to set aside a special day each week when missionaries can rest from the day-to-day labors of missionary work, prepare for the week to come, and perform any necessary chores.

Preparation Day

Preparation day, or P-day, is a multi-faceted day. It is a day that is not just a luxury to look forward to, but a physical and spiritual necessity. The purpose of P-day is to prepare temporally for the coming week, to rest from your labors of the past week, rejuvenate your body and spirit so you have the necessary energy to get through the week ahead, and to cultivate meaningful leisure experiences while on your mission. All of this before heading out the door for an evening of proselyting!

Preparation day does not officially begin until after all the required morning activities are completed. Therefore, P-day should begin just like every other day on your mission – wake-up at the same time, 30 minutes of exercise, individual and companionship study, breakfast, etc. After completing the usual morning routine, the remainder of the day, until after dinner, is yours to spend how you and your companion decide. However, it would be wise to spend it completing necessary chores, preparing for the next week, and participating in leisure activities that will take your mind off the day-to-day routine of missionary work.

Most missionaries will have a desire to participate in leisure activities that allow them to see and explore their mission, especially if they are serving in a foreign land. You should visit cultural and historical sites, libraries, museums, art galleries, shopping centers, outdoor parks, hiking trails, and even participate in sporting activities on P-day. Remember to only participate in activities that have been approved by your mission president. He understands the mission and knows of any dangers or pitfalls associated with certain activities and events. Follow his inspired guidance and you will be blessed with protection. Also, be aware that many of the activities you may choose to participate in can be time-consuming and exhausting. Make sure you plan accordingly in order to get all the necessary chores and preparations done for the coming week to ensure your temporal needs are met.

Take advantage of the time you have to rest whether it is on the Sabbath Day, on Preparation Day, or both. After experiencing a day... or two of rest, you will be refreshed and ready to serve with all your heart, might, mind, and strength for another week.

RECOVERY FROM EXERCISE

When following any exercise program, there is a tendency to do too-much, too-soon, especially in the beginning. Resist the temptation to do this. Instead progress slowly and gradually. You need to lay a solid foundation for your body before it is ready to handle more stress. This can take some time, so be patient.

If you do not lay this critical foundation, your body may have a tendency to succumb to over-training easier, increasing your risk of injury, pain, discomfort, soreness, illness, and failure. Unfortunately, this will prevent you from benefiting from the exercise program and may, in fact, harm you even more. If this occurs, or if you experience periods of illness or injury, it is recommended that you take a short break from your daily exercise program. Typically, the time-off should be limited to one week, and in most cases, only three or four days are sufficient to fully recover and return back to normal.

When the Twelve Apostles returned to Jesus

following their assignments to preach, teach, and heal the people where they served, Jesus patiently listened to their stories and then wisely said to them, "Come ye yourselves apart into a desert place, and rest a while" (Mark 6:31). Jesus understood from personal experience how physically and spiritually exhausting it is to serve in a full-time capacity. Therefore, He required His apostles to rest often to restore their health and energy before going out among the people again. Just as Jesus required His apostles to rest, you too are expected to rest in order to maintain your health and restore your energy. Doing so can help you continue serving to your full potential.

OVERCOMING THE NATURAL MAN

A mission is a critical time in your life. It is during this time that you begin to establish and strengthen your own ideas, values, beliefs, and lifestyle habits that you will embrace for the rest of your life. Your mission becomes the basis for some very real, life-changing decisions. During this time you will, perhaps, form your beliefs and habits related to health and fitness. You have the choice to either develop healthy or unhealthy lifestyle habits. You can choose to be healthy and thrive on your mission and throughout your life, or you can choose to succumb to the temptations of the natural man and experience health-related problems making it difficult to handle the challenges of a mission and everyday life.

To perform at your best, free from sickness, disease, and injury while on your mission, you need to learn how to overcome the natural man. Either you will overcome the natural man, or the natural man will overcome you. It is your choice. At times it may seem difficult and even impossible to overcome the natural man, but, in fact, it is possible and even essential because the natural man is an enemy to God (see Mosiah 3:19). However, it does take a measure of self-discipline and commitment to achieve it as King Benjamin explained: "For the natural man is an enemy to God, and has been from the fall of Adam, and will be, forever and ever, unless he yields to the enticings of the Holy Spirit, and putteth off the natural man and becometh a saint through the atonement of Christ the Lord, and becometh as a child, submissive, meek, humble, patient, full of love, willing to submit to all things which the Lord seeth fit to inflict upon him, even as a child doth submit to his father" (Mosiah 3:19). Once you keep and embrace this commitment the benefits will far outweigh the sacrifice involved.

Unfortunately, mission life provides a number of obstacles that the natural man can exploit if you allow them to take hold in your life. These obstacles can be relatively easy to overcome once you have recognized them and implemented the necessary strategies to change them. The most common obstacles affecting a healthy missionary life are: too much stress, not enough time, a lack of energy, no motivation, and idolatry. Following is an explanation of each with some strategies to help you overcome them.

TO MUCH STRESS

Perhaps the most common and valid of all the obstacles afflicting missionaries is too much stress. Stress is a very real response to the demands of everyday missionary life. Undoubtedly, the process of saving souls is extremely difficult and arduous. Add to that the other aspects of missionary life that result in stress, such as following a demanding schedule, constantly changing areas, companions, and responsibilities; and being separated from family and friends and you have an extremely stress-filled environment.

Essentially, there are two types of stress that can arise from any one of several sources. The two types of stress are positive and negative stress. Positive stress is actually a good and desirable thing. This type of stress still places demands and burdens on the body and mind, but it will also lead to feelings of excitement and joy. Physical exercise and an increase in leadership responsibilities are examples of positive stress. Negative stress is disturbing and depressing. It has the greatest impact on the body in a damaging way. Although negative stress may sometimes be out of your control, the way you handle it is not out of your control. By conditioning your body to cope with its demands, and reacting in a positive manner, you can do a lot to prevent its harmful side-effects.

The sources that each of these stresses can come from are environmental, nutritional, physical, emotional, and mental. Environmental factors relate to the geographic area where you live, the conditions of your environment (noise, air quality, etc.) and the people you associate with in that environment. Nutritional factors relate to the quality, type, and amount of food and beverages you consume. The physical factors include illnesses, diseases, injuries, accidents, physical exercise, toxic waste accumulation, pregnancy, and growth spurts. Emotional factors stem from abuse, death or illness of a loved one, increase in responsibility, phobias, and fears. Mental factors include things such as learning, understanding, and memorizing new things like a foreign language or a scripture verse.

The real issue is not so much that you have stress, because most things in life will cause some level of stress, but rather, how you manage stress when it does come. The more effectively you can manage the stress in your life, the more successful you can be at serving a mission. Here are some proven strategies for effectively managing stress:

Increase Faith and Trust in Jesus Christ
Stress has a unique way of amplifying the areas in your life that may be weak or which you are struggling with. For example, if you have an impaired immune

system from a result of poor nutritional habits, then, even the smallest amount of stress might cause you to become sick.

Fortunately, we have been promised that if we grow closer to Christ and have faith in Him during times of stress, then weak areas will become stronger. Jesus said, "I give unto men weakness that they may be humble...for if they humble themselves before me, and have faith in me, then will I make weak things become strong unto them" (Ether 12:27). During times of stress true peace will come from having faith and trust in Jesus Christ as the Savior and Redeemer of the world. The stronger your faith and trust in Jesus, the stronger you will be the next time stress comes and the better you will be at coping with it.

Plan and Prepare for Change

Very few things in mission life remain stable. Change is something you can depend on. Your environment, areas, companions, and contacts are always changing. Despite the constant change, proper planning and preparation can reduce stress and anxiety. When you have properly planned and prepared for something, you are better suited to handle the changes that will come.

You can prepare for the stress of mission life by studying the history, customs, cultures, traditions, and cuisines of your mission and surrounding area before leaving home. Talk to return missionaries who have served in the same mission to learn more about the missionary lifestyle in that part of the world. The more you know and understand about your mission and what to expect before leaving, the less anxiety and stress you will experience.

Exercise Regularly and Eat Healthy

Exercise can improve your mood. Chemicals known as endorphins flood the brain during exercise. These endorphins decrease pain and increase relaxation, lifting your spirit and making you feel good. Exercise gives you energy and a sense of accomplishment. It also helps you breathe more deeply. This causes your lymph system to be stimulated, detoxifying your body and sending a flow of oxygen into tissues and organs. Stimulation of the lymph system triggers a relaxation response throughout the body decrease stressful feelings.

Proper nutrition provides the body with the right combination of vitamins, minerals, and nutrients which, in turn, gives the body more energy. Fueling the body with the right nutrients allows the body to repair itself while strengthening the immune system, keeping illness and disease at bay.

Rest and Relax Sufficiently

It is important for the body to get sufficient amounts of rest and sleep. The human body is designed to function optimally when it gets enough rest each and every day. It needs that time to repair and restore itself. In addition to resting, it is important to learn to relax and enjoy life by participating in meaningful leisure time. Participate in activities that refresh you physically and emotionally. This may include playing a musical instrument, reading, doing something artistic, visiting a museum or other historical places, or participating in a physical activity. Figure out what helps you relax and spend adequate time doing it.

Have a Positive Attitude

Your reaction to any given event or situation can increase or decrease the amount of stress you experience. Even when you do not have control over the situation, you can still control your reaction to it. You can also control your overall outlook and attitude toward your mission experience. The way you respond to the stress that comes into your life may be an indicator to the strength of your testimony of the gospel of Jesus Christ, not because you handle every situation perfectly, but because in the midst of the stressful situation, you recognize your natural weakness and rely on the Lord for help and guidance to assist and comfort you in your time of need.

NOT ENOUGH TIME

The biggest obstacle for some missionaries is they just do not have the extra time to spend on taking care of their health needs while on their mission. There is no doubt that the daily schedule for missionaries is rigid and demanding with very little free time. In fact, not long ago a lack of time was a very real and valid concern for missionaries. Although the Missionary "White" Handbook instructed missionaries to schedule time each day for exercise (*Missionary Handbook, 17*), in reality there was very little, if any, free time to accomplish this while continuing to follow the other required items on the schedule.

Fortunately, in recent years, church leaders have thoughtfully included 30 minutes of exercise time in the daily missionary schedule. Following are some strategies on how to make the most of this time while accomplishing all of your health, fitness, and nutrition needs.

Plan and Prepare

Every meeting and activity you participate in during your mission is typically scheduled, planned-out, and prepared in advance. You should follow this same approach for each of your workouts and meals. The weekly-scheduled planning session is an ideal time to do this. You should plan the exercises you will be including in your workouts and the food you will be including in your meals for the following week. Document this information in your weekly planner or in the *Missionary Fitness Journal*, available free at www.missionaryfitness.com. By planning and preparing these things in advance you will not waste valuable time deciding which exercises you should do or which food you should eat each and every day.

Exercise First Thing in the Morning

The best time of day to exercise is shortly after waking up in the morning. Coincidentally, according to the daily schedule, missionaries are instructed to exercise first thing in the morning. Exercising at this time wakes the body up and gives you more energy during the day allowing you to be more productive. You are also much better prepared to handle the pressures and responsibilities of the day if you exercise before these things begin to pile up.

Multi-task

Another way to make the most of your time is to multi-task. Multi-tasking is performing more than one activity at the same time. Multi-tasking is not for everyone. It requires some skill and possibly even a degree of coordination. You may find that certain activities on your mission are more conducive to multi-tasking than others. Some of the best times during the day to multi-task are while exercising and eating. During these times you can read or listen to the scriptures, pray, meditate, write in your journal, or make phone calls to schedule appointments. Your imagination is the only limit in figuring out what you can do to multi-task at these times.

LACK OF ENERGY

The fatigue factor is another problem for missionaries at some point during their mission. Poor nutrition, insufficient sleep, and inactivity can all cause you to have a lack of energy. The following are some strategies that will help you increase your energy levels while on your mission.

Exercise Everyday

Exercise everyday except Sunday. Exercise recharges energy levels and increases alertness and productivity. Exercise increases blood flow allowing you to get more oxygen to the muscles and organs of your body, especially your brain giving you more energy.

Follow a Healthy Nutritional Plan

A lack of vitamins, minerals, and other nutrients leads to a malnourished body. The body has to slow its metabolism and other physiological processes to make up for the lack of nutrition. When you eat a healthy, well-balanced diet, the body receives all the necessary nutrients to perform optimally, providing the energy necessary to sustain you throughout the day.

Get Sufficient Sleep Each Night

The body needs time to recharge, repair, and restore itself. It is free to do this at night while you are sleeping. If you do not give your body the sleep it needs, it can not fully recover, leaving you too tired to perform your missionary duties.

NO MOTIVATION

With so much going on in your life as a missionary and having several obstacles to halt your progress, it can sometimes be difficult to find the motivation to live a healthy lifestyle. The following are a few ways to stay motivated during your mission.

Be Consistent

It is much easier to follow and maintain a daily exercise and healthy eating program after you have been following one consistently for a period of time. Be consistent and put a little effort in maintaining your health on a day-to-day basis. As you do so, your motivation level will increase.

Document Your Progress

Record the details of your workouts, meals, and sleep. This can be done by using your weekly planner or the *Missionary Fitness Journal*, available free at www.missionaryfitness.com. Documenting this information is vital in knowing where you started, how far you have come, and how far you may still need to go in relation to the goals you have set for yourself. It is always inspiring to see how far you have come and what you have accomplished. As you observe your progress you will continue to be motivated.

Get Your Companion Involved

One of the best ways to stay motivated and accountable in accomplishing anything is to get another person involved. Some missionaries will do just fine exercising and eating right on their own. However, other missionaries may need the added support and motivation that another person can offer. If this is the case with you, your companion can be a great asset. You should get him involved in whatever capacity you can. He can provide support, accountability, and most of all, motivation.

Prepare the Night Before

Each night you should lay out your exercise clothes beside your bed. As soon as your alarm goes off in the morning put them on and immediately begin your workout. The sooner you put them on, the more motivated you will be to exercise.

BEWARE OF IDOLATRY

Certainly giving up the comforts and lifestyle you enjoyed before missionary service and sacrificing 18 or 24-months of your life to serve God should be sufficient enough evidence that you are not an offender of idolatry. In fact, on the surface it appears that missionary life is the antithesis of idolatry. Unfortunately, simply being a missionary does not guarantee protection from falling victim to idolatry.

The word idolatry comes from the Greek word eidololatria meaning "image" or "figure worship." Our Father in Heaven has specifically said, "Thou shalt have no other gods before me. Thou shalt not make unto thee any graven image, or any likeness of any thing that is in heaven above, or that is in the earth beneath, or that is in the water under the earth: Thou shalt not bow down thyself to them, nor serve them: for I the Lord thy God am a jealous God" (Exodus 20:3-5). In its simplest form, idolatry is giving honor, praise, and worship to someone or something other than the true and living God.

The most notable mention of idolatry in scriptures comes when Moses took longer on Mount Sinai than the Israelites expected, leaving them restless. They "gathered themselves together unto Aaron, and said unto him...make us gods, which shall go before us." And Aaron made a molten calf, and the people said, "These be thy gods, O Israel, which brought thee up out of the land of Egypt" (Exodus 32:1, 4).

The Children of Israel never thought about denouncing God when they persuaded Aaron to make a golden calf. Professed reverence for the true and living God and actual idolatry are perfectly compatible and are often performed concurrently. In this instance the golden calf was not set up as a rival with God, but under the pretense of being a help or a stepping stone to worshipping Him. Nevertheless in doing so, a great sin was committed. The honor that should have been given to God was, instead, given to a graven image.

Even though idolatry today is similar to the idolatry of the ancient Israelites in blending reverence for the true God with the worship of images and idols, it is much less obvious and sometimes more difficult to recognize. The more sophisticated, modern forms of idolatry no longer take on the appearance of a golden calf. They are much more subtle and can unknowingly take hold of your life threatening to weaken or corrupt your faith and testimony. The most relevant example of this form of idolatry, in regards to the subject at hand, is an obsessed fixation on the pursuit of physical beauty and optimal health. Although your body is literally a temple of the Holy Spirit and you have a stewardship to care for it, you should not make your appearance, physical fitness, nutrition, or health a source of worship.

As you begin to pursue a healthier life by implementing the principles learned in this book, you will soon discover changes with your physical body that you may never have experienced before. Typically these changes are positive and are a great source of motivation to continue caring for your physical health and appearance. Unfortunately, in some instances these changes can ignite unhealthy, idolatrous behavior. After experiencing the benefits from the new and positive changes, there may be a tendency for some missionaries to be overly consumed with their physical fitness, appearance, nutrition, and health in order to maintain the new look and feel.

The apostle Paul had witnessed this type of behavior during his ministry among the Greeks and Romans and saw how detrimental it could be to a person. At this time in history, these cultures took great pride in their physical appearance and athletic skills. They would spend a large majority of their time engaged in activities to enhance these attributes. This behavior concerned Paul because it kept the people from progressing spiritually. Paul wanted these people to realize there was more to life than just the physical body. He wanted them to recognize the primary importance of the spirit. In reflecting on these experiences, Paul included the following statement in his letter to Timothy, "For bodily exercise profiteth little: but godliness is profitable unto all things, having promise of the life that now is, and of that which is to come" (1 Timothy 4:8).

Paul was very clear in his wording when he made this statement. He did not say that exercise is a waste of time and should not be performed. He simply explained that engaging in exercise and physical activity is not as beneficial as seeking after righteousness. He taught that more blessings would come through developing the spirit than through developing the body. He emphasized that obtaining eternal life is predicated on the spiritual pursuits more than the physical pursuits.

If you have put your physical pursuits ahead of your spiritual pursuits, then you may be guilty of idolatry. Thankfully, as with most transgressions, idolatry can be overcome. The Children of Israel were finally able to forsake this great sin. They nearly rooted it out during their 40 years wandering in the wilderness, but were not completely successful until abandoning it during the Babylonian exile.

Fortunately, you do not need to wander in a

wilderness for 40 years or be exiled from your home or mission to achieve freedom from the obsession of physical health and beauty. Any idolatrous tendency can be abandoned by following the teachings of the One who provides salvation to all. Jesus taught, "...If any man will come after me, let him deny himself, and take up his cross, and follow me. For whosoever will save his life shall lose it: and whosoever will lose his life for my sake shall find it. For what is a man profited, if he shall gain the whole world, and lose his own soul? or what shall a man give in exchange for his soul" (Matthew 16:24-26)? Jesus taught that for a man to take up his cross and overcome any selfish desires, he needed to deny himself of all ungodliness and every worldly lust and keep the commandments (see JST Matthew 16:26).

Heavenly Father and Jesus Christ should be the central focus of your life and your worship. As a missionary, you should only be concerned with your health, nutrition, fitness, and appearance only to the extent they enable you to be a better missionary and help you serve the Lord more effectively on your mission.

SET REALISTIC GOALS

Besides the strategies mentioned above, another way to overcome the natural man while on your mission and throughout your life is the simple practice of setting realistic goals. Setting goals will serve you well while you are serving.

Just as you set spiritual and proselyting goals as a missionary, you should also set physical goals. Having a clear picture of where you are going in regards to your physical health will give you the mental edge and motivation to overcome temptations that may cause you to give in to the natural man and fall victim to the common obstacles mentioned earlier.

If you are totally committed to developing healthy lifestyle habits while on your mission, you need to set some very specific and realistic long-term and short-term goals. Developing clear and concise goals will help you stay focused and committed to maintaining your health and fitness while on your mission.

There are a few things to remember when setting goals. It can be overwhelming when changing lifestyle habits and establishing new ones, so be patient and realistic in accomplishing them. Trying to do too much, too soon will only cause discouragement and keep you from accomplishing your goals. Isaiah speaks of this patience when he said, "precept upon precept; line upon line; here a little, and there a little" (Isaiah 28:10).

Focus on progress, not perfection. Developing a healthy lifestyle is a lifetime endeavor. It is a process that should become a part of life. You will make mistakes and you will fall short every once-in-awhile. Do not be overly hard on yourself, too critical, or get discouraged. Doing so will only sabotage your ability to accomplish your goals and may halt your progress.

Set realistic goals that are specific and time-sensitive. Do not set them so low that you do not need to work hard to accomplish them. On the other hand, do not set them so high that you have no chance of accomplishing them. If you set your goals too high and consistently fail to achieve them, you may become discouraged. After accomplishing a goal, immediately set a new one. In setting this new goal, make it a little more challenging, but keep it realistic.

Clearly, life as a missionary does not make you immune to the temptations of the natural man. However, as you strive to overcome the common obstacles to living a healthy lifestyle and commit to setting realistic goals, you will be blessed in your ability to overcome the natural man.

You will increase in spiritual and physical strength and you "shall mount up with wings as eagles; [and] shall run, and not be weary; and...shall walk, and not faint" (see Isaiah 40:31).

GOING THE EXTRA MILE

Jesus has always encouraged everyone to do more than the bare minimum when He proclaimed during the Sermon on the Mount, "And whosoever shall compel thee to go a mile, go with him twain" (Matthew 5:41). At the time Jesus gave this sermon, Judea was under Roman law. One of the many laws the Romans compelled the Jews to follow permitted a Roman soldier to command any Jewish man or boy nearby to carry his armor, weapons, packs, or any other burden the soldier would otherwise have to carry himself. Being more civilized than other armies, the Romans limited this task to just one Roman mile. A Roman mile was a measure of 1,000 paces, each pace consisting of approximately five feet, making the Roman mile slightly shorter than the mile we know of today, which is 5,280 feet.

Such recruitment is best illustrated during Jesus' walk from the city of Jerusalem up to Calvary Hill where He was to be crucified. After Jesus collapsed under the heavy weight of carrying His own cross, the Roman soldiers who were ushering Him along, grabbed a man out of the crowd, making him carry the cross the remaining distance (see Matthew 27:32). By some estimates, this remaining distance was approximately 1,000 paces.

No Jewish man or boy liked being forced to carry anything, any distance for a Roman soldier. Surely they were anxious to drop the load as soon as they counted off the thousandth step. Few people will do more than what is expected. Jesus knew and taught that it is only when people voluntarily give more than required, that they receive greater blessings. This is why Jesus said if someone compelled you to carry their load for one mile, then you should go two miles instead.

As a missionary, you will learn and apply this principle in many aspects of your life; in teaching, preaching, baptizing, blessing, and serving others, but have you learned to apply this principle to your physical health?

Too often people measure out exactly what is expected of them and do just the minimum required - going the first mile - and nothing more. Most people already know how to go the first mile as it relates to their health. After all, you could not live very long without doing so. The first mile of physical health is essentially what you must do just to maintain life - like breathing, eating, drinking fluids, and sleeping. With the hectic pace of mission life, missionaries tend to only go the "first mile" in regards to their physical health. Unfortunately, this can lead to health problems and sometimes even injuries.

Fortunately, Jesus taught there is a better way when he said to go the extra mile. He was saying to do more than the bare minimum, more than is required or expected. The first mile you carry the burden because you are made to, because it is expected of you. The second mile you carry the burden because you choose to. During the first mile you were the oppressed. During the second mile you are equal to the oppressor. The oppressor has no power over you on the second mile. It is during the second mile where you begin to truly learn about yourself and when you begin to see the real blessings of living a physically healthy and active lifestyle. The extra mile turns the ordinary into the extraordinary, the expected into the unexpected.

You go the extra mile for your health when you do an extra repetition, an extra set, add an extra exercise, when you politely decline the offer for a second helping of food or dessert, or when you order the healthy alternative at the restaurant. The extra mile turns responsibility into opportunity. When you go the extra mile your attitude shifts from "have to" to "want to."

Another part of going the extra mile means bearing one another's burdens. This is the kind of life a disciple of Christ should lead. You should live a life of willing submission to those things that are beneficial to you as well as others, to your own health and the health of others. Going the extra mile means to be an example to others, to share your knowledge and understanding of the physical body and the importance of maintaining its health. Remember the principles you learn as you read this book. Share them with your companions, the people in the area you serve, and your family once you return home. Teach others how living a healthy lifestyle has helped you become a better missionary and servant of God. Then show them how they too can transform their bodies and spirits as you did.

With some practice, going the extra mile will become an effortless habit and it will improve every aspect of your life, including your health. Sadly, you will find that the second mile is not very crowded and it can sometimes be lonely. Jesus led a lonely life as He accomplished infinitely more for mankind than what was expected of Him. He obeyed Heavenly Father perfectly to fulfill the law. He willingly submitted to the agonizing pain in the Garden of Gethsemane and accepted the death penalty on the cross to atone for everyone's sins. He went the extra mile to provide forgiveness and eternal life for all. On your mission and throughout the rest of your life, you must go the extra mile, not because you grudgingly have to, but because you freely and gladly want to, out of love for Jesus and Heavenly Father for the many gifts they have lovingly given you.

CONCLUSION:

Maintaining Your Body and Spirit for Life

As your mission draws to a close, thoughts of home and of the "real world" will begin to creep slowly into your mind. At this time you will begin to realize that it has been an extremely rare privilege for you to have gone to the area of the world you were chosen to labor. You will have had the privilege to experience a different culture, different people, different way of life, different foods, different customs, and maybe even a different language. You will have amassed a long list of fond memories and special experiences as you have served. You will look back over your time of service and realize that you have also learned many things about yourself. Your testimony of the Savior will have grown, your knowledge of the gospel and the scriptures will have more than likely increased, and you will probably have abandoned many bad habits, only to replace them with good ones.

As you return home you will notice the many ways you have grown and matured as things that once appealed to you before, no longer appeal to you. Your life will take on a whole new meaning and direction. You will now be more focused on the things that really matter in life, the things that have eternal significance. The weeks and months of adjustment following a mission are difficult and complicated at best, but are nonetheless critical to the success of a healthy and joyful life. Despite all the many changes you will encounter after returning home, perhaps the most difficult part of the adjustment period is learning to maintain the good habits and behaviors you developed while serving so faithfully.

As a missionary you will be challenged to develop and master certain habits and behaviors which are based on eternal principles and laws. You will have had the opportunity to transform your body and spirit while you served the Lord. Unfortunately, the benefits of this transformation do not last. You must continue to nurture and participate in the habits and behaviors that allowed for this transformation to occur. It is a lifelong pursuit, one that must continue after your mission.

Once you return home and let go of the intense missionary schedule, you may also be tempted to let go of some of these fundamental habits you developed as a result of living such a schedule. Of these habits, there is a few that if continued to be practiced once at home, will bring you the same physical and spiritual health, joy, and success experienced on a mission. These habits are regular prayer, daily scripture and gospel study, daily service, and daily physical maintenance.

REGULAR PRAYER

Communicating with Heavenly Father frequently gives you strength and power to continue steadfastly in your missionary work. The more you pray the stronger and more faithful you will become. During a mission you pray constantly, both individually and as a companionship, with investigators and members, at meetings, and prior to every meal. Each morning you begin the day with prayer, individually and as a companionship. This process is repeated at the end of the day before going to bed as well. You pray before studying, before leaving your apartment, and whenever you need direction in your missionary efforts or personal life.

Frequent, consistent prayer will continue to keep you strong and faithful after returning home from your mission. Whether it is for guidance with a career choice, direction with whom you should marry, or help with your studies in school, you should always seek the Lord for both spiritual and temporal assistance. Pray regularly, several times a day. Pray continuously in your heart, offering up thanks for blessings, appeals for forgiveness, and strength when temptation is near.

DAILY SCRIPTURE AND GOSPEL STUDY

Every single morning on your mission you have the opportunity to study the gospel individually and with a companion. This habit keeps the doctrines and principles of the gospel fresh in your mind and helps strengthen you against the adversary's grasp. It also leads to an increase in faith and spiritual strength.

After returning home from your mission, you will no longer have a companion to hold you accountable for scripture and gospel study. This means you must be motivated and disciplined enough to maintain the practice on your own. You may find the best way to stay motivated and disciplined is by continuing to read and study the scriptures early in the morning, just as you did on your mission, before the pressures and worries of the day come upon you. Doing this allows you to be more receptive to communication from the Holy Spirit and it opens up the way to commune with your Heavenly Father. Another way to stay motivated and disciplined is to invite family members, friends, or your spouse (once you are married) to read and study together. They will take the place of your missionary companions providing insight and understanding you may not have been able to receive on your own.

Another great way to continue your scripture and gospel study is to participate in the Church Educational System. As soon as possible after returning home from your mission, you would be well-advised to enroll in an institute of religion class at your local college or university. This formal study will allow you to learn the doctrines of the Kingdom of God and increase your understanding of the gospel. It is also a great way to interact and socialize with other like-minded individuals.

Scripture and gospel study should include writing down your thoughts, feelings, and impressions in a journal. Just as you document the physical aspects of your life in your *Missionary Fitness Journal*, available free at www.missionaryfitness.com, you should also document the spiritual aspects of your life in another journal.

It will be a great privilege for you to be able to look back in your journal and relive the many experiences that you have enjoyed throughout your life. There is a saying that goes, "if you do not write it down, it did not happen." Of course this saying is not literally true. However, it does stress the fact that, in many cases, it is nearly impossible to remember the details of significant events that have occurred in your life. If you write these events down daily in a journal, along with your thoughts and feelings about them, you will be more confident in remembering the events of your life. Essentially, journal writing provides an insurance of sorts on your memory, or lack thereof.

DAILY SERVICE

One of the keys to quickly adapting to regular life after returning home from your mission is by continuing to serve. By serving others you will be able to persistently build up a wall of protection against the evils of the world that would have you stumble and fall. As a missionary you have the opportunity to regularly serve others. You are given several opportunities each day to serve. Look for opportunities to serve after returning home. These opportunities may not be as obvious to you or may not come as readily to you as they do when on a mission, but if you seek for them, they will come. Remember, when you are in the service of your fellow beings you are only in the service of your God (see Mosiah 2:17).

When you return home and are officially released as a missionary, let your Stake President and Bishop know that you are ready to receive a calling as soon as possible. However, do not wait for a formal invitation or calling before helping or serving others. Be eager, willing, and even volunteer to pray in meetings, go home teaching, bless or pass the sacrament, and help those in need. Immediately become involved in church and quorum activities, service projects, and fellowshipping others. This will allow for the many service opportunities to present themselves to you.

Service also includes sharing your testimony with others, which can strengthen them in the gospel or even bring them to the gospel. You never know what your words can do to impact the life of the one who hears them. You already know how to share your testimony. As a missionary you do it several times a day. Pray and look for opportunities to continue to share your testimony upon returning home.

Temple attendance is another way to serve after returning home. The vicarious work you have the privilege of performing will eternally bless the people you serve and will allow you the opportunity to ponder the things in life that are truly important. This allows you to find answers to troubling questions or to simply feel a little needed peace.

DAILY PHYSICAL MAINTENANCE

The physical habits you develop on your mission are just as crucial as the spiritual habits. The way you look and the way you feel physically will have a profound affect on every other aspect of your life. After returning home you should continue to participate in some sort of physical activity everyday. As you maintain this habit you will strengthen your body and it will be able to perform day-to-day tasks more efficiently. You will have a better respect for the eternal nature of your body, which, in turn, will allow you to make wise choices regarding the things you put into it, the things you do to it, and the things you do with it.

Continue to follow all the healthy habits you established on your mission as well. As you have learned, fueling your body with the right nutrients and resting from your labors can go a long way in keeping your body and spirit healthy and clean.

Part of maintaining your physical body includes maintaining the appearance and grooming standards you follow as a missionary. After returning home, continue to represent the Lord by keeping a neat and well-groomed appearance. Consider the words of a disappointed prophet after observing the lack of grooming habits from some returned missionaries:

"I want you to know it is hard for me to be disappointed...But a few things disappoint me occasionally and one of them is the returned missionary who, after two years of taking great pride in how he looks and what he represents, returns to campus or some other place to see how quickly he can let his hair grow, how fully he can develop a moustache and long sideburns and push to the very margins of appropriate grooming, how clumpy his shoes [can] get, how tattered his clothes,...how close to being grubby he can get...

"Please, you returned missionaries...please do not abandon in appearance or principle or habit the great experiences of the mission field...we do not expect you to wear a tie, white shirt, and a dark blue suit every day...But surely it is not too much to ask you that your grooming be maintained, that your personal habits reflect cleanliness and dignity and pride in the principles of the gospel you taught. We ask you for the good of the kingdom and all those who have done and yet do take pride in you" (Kimball, 593).

Read this book as often as you need before you leave on your mission, while you are serving, and after you have returned home in order to remember the eternal principles it contains. These principles will not only assist you in transforming your body and spirit while you serve, but will also assist you in maintaining your body and spirit long after you have returned home from your mission.

Your mission is a stepping stone to greater physical and spiritual health. It is only the beginning of a whole new life. As you transform your body and spirit while you serve, you have entered in by the gate to the rest of your life. Nephi explains it best:

"Wherefore, do the things which I have told you I have seen that your Lord and your Redeemer should do; for, for this cause have they been shown unto me, that ye might know the gate by which ye should enter... And then are ye in this straight and narrow path that leads to eternal life; yea, ye have entered in by the gate; ye have done according to the commandments of the Father and the Son; and ye have received the Holy Ghost, which witnesses of the Father and the Son, unto the fulfilling of the promise which he hath made, that if ye entered in by the way ye should receive. And now, my beloved brethren, after ye have gotten into this strait and narrow path, I would ask if all is done? Behold, I say unto you, Nay; for ye have not come thus far save it were by the word of Christ with unshaken faith in him, relying wholly upon the merits of him who is mighty to save. Wherefore, ye must press forward with a steadfastness in Christ, having a perfect brightness of hope, and a love of God and of all men. Wherefore, if ye shall press forward, feasting upon the word of Christ, and endure to the end, behold, thus saith the Father: Ye shall have eternal life. And now, behold, my beloved brethren, this is the way; and there is none other way nor name given under heaven whereby man can be saved in the kingdom of God. And now, behold, this is the doctrine of Christ, and the only and true doctrine of the Father, and of the Son, and of the Holy Ghost, which is one God, without end" (2 Nephi 31: 17-21).

Continue to be active in fulfilling God's purposes. Glorify Him in your body and spirit (see 1 Corinthians 6:20). Do not settle for anything less than what Heavenly Father expects from you, than what you expect from yourself, than what you deserve as a returned missionary and as a child of God. Do not underestimate your potential to transform your life and the lives of those around you. As you prepare your body and spirit for service and subsequently maintain it after you have returned home, God will bless you and He will be with you always. Remember, the Lord loves and blesses His returned missionaries.

For further help and resources in preparing your body and spirit for service and for maintaining your body and spirit after your mission, please visit www.missionaryfitness.com and check out the products and services that will complement your healthy and faithful lifestyle.

Bibliography

Ballard, M. Russell. "The Greatest Generation of Missionaries," *Ensign*, November 2002: 47.

Bednar, David A. "Becoming a Missionary," *Ensign*, November 2005: 45.

Benson, Ezra Taft. "Third Day Afternoon Meeting," *Official Report of the One Hundred Fortieth Annual General Conference of The Church of Jesus Christ of Latter-day Saints* (Salt Lake City: The Church of Jesus Christ of Latter-day Saints, April 1970).

Benson, Ezra Taft. "To the 'Youth of the Noble Birthright," *Ensign*, May 1986: 45.

Cooper, Kenneth. *Faith-Based Fitness* (Nashville: Thomas Nelson, Inc., 1995).

Doty, Donald B. "Missionary Health Preparation," *Ensign*, March 2007: 63.

Hinckley, Richard G. *Mission President Homecoming* (Arlington Hills Ward, Federal Heights Stake Center, July 11, 2004).

Intellectual Reserve, Inc. *Missionary Handbook* (Salt Lake City: The Church of Jesus Christ of Latter-day Saints, 1990).

Kimball, Spencer W. *The Teachings of Spencer W. Kimball* (West Valley City: Bookcraft, Inc., 1982).

Kimball, Spencer W. "When the World Will Be Converted," *Ensign*, October 1974: 7-8.

McConkie, Bruce R. *Mormon Doctrine* (West Valley City: Bookcraft, Inc., 1966).

McConkie, Bruce R. *The Mortal Messiah*: From Bethlehem to Calvary, Book 1 (Salt Lake City: Deseret Book Company, 1979).

McKay, David O. "The 'Whole' Man," *Improvement Era*, April 1952: 221.

Smith, Hyrum M. & Sjodahl, Janne M. *Doctrine and Covenants Commentary* (Salt Lake City: Deseret Book Company, 1978)

Smith, Joseph F. *Eighty-third Semi-Annual Conference of The Church of Jesus Christ of Latter-day Saints* (Salt Lake City: The Deseret News, Oct 1912).

The Church of Jesus Christ of Latter-day Saints General Handbook of Instructions, No. 20 (Salt Lake City: The First Presidency of The Church of Jesus Christ of Latter-day Saints, 1968).

About the Author

Calvin Buhler is a leading expert in the field of health, nutrition, and human performance. He is the founder of several successful health and fitness companies and is an exercise and nutrition consultant for elite athletes, business leaders, sports teams, nutritional supplement companies, and fitness equipment manufacturers. Buhler helps individuals and organizations reach higher levels of performance and success by implementing universal principles and strategies gleaned from years of education, research, and experience.

Buhler is a highly sought after speaker, writer, and consultant providing training, education, and instruction throughout the world. Known as a dynamic speaker, Buhler's style is informative and inspirational. In addition to authoring books and training materials for clients, he has also written several articles for online and print media. He has made frequent radio appearances and has been a member of the advisory board for several nutritional supplement companies.

Buhler's love for health began at a young age growing up as the son and grandson of medical doctors. A love for exercise and nutrition soon followed during his competitive years as an athlete. Buhler's highly-decorated athletic career culminated in achieving NCAA All-American status and winning the prized NSCA's All-American Athlete of the Year award. He still trains and competes as a way of staying in-shape and leading by example. Buhler holds a Bachelor of Science degree in Health and Exercise Science and is a Certified Strength and Conditioning Specialist with the National Strength and Conditioning Association.

Following an outstanding academic and athletic career, Buhler was called to serve a 2-year mission for The Church of Jesus Christ of Latter-day Saints. While serving his mission, he held callings as a trainer, District Leader, Zone Leader, and Assistant to the President. He was part of the first group of missionaries to pilot the "Preach My Gospel" program. He also provided valuable input regarding the addition of 30-minutes to the daily missionary schedule for physical exercise.

www.ingramcontent.com/pod-product-compliance
Lightning Source LLC
LaVergne TN
LVHW011227080426
835509LV00005B/360